Let's talk about preparing for your baby's birth

Disclaimer

This book and the techniques and information within it are not intended
to replace medical care from qualified healthcare professionals. It is a
general guide to your options and choices, enabling you to discuss your
wishes in detail with your midwife/doctor. The author and publisher
cannot accept responsibility for readers' personal decisions about which
techniques and information they use during birth.

The book is aimed at women with straightforward pregnancies.
Women with more complex needs during pregnancy and labour may find
that they have a different balance of benefits and risks.

Please note that illustrations are for general information and are not
anatomically precise.

While the author trained with the National Childbirth Trust (NCT),
this book is in no way affiliated with, authorised by or endorsed by the
NCT.

All MP3s can be accessed here: www.baby-bumps.net/bookmp3s

Let's talk about preparing for your baby's birth

Jackie Kietz

pinter & martin

Let's talk about preparing for your baby's birth

First published in the UK by Pinter & Martin Ltd 2020

Copyright © Jackie Kietz 2020
Chapter twenty © Kate Cameron 2020

All rights reserved

ISBN 978-1-78066-700-3

Also available as an ebook

The right of Jackie Kietz to be identified as the author of this work
has been asserted by her in accordance with the Copyright, Designs
and Patent Act of 1988

Edited by Susan Last
Index by Helen Bilton
Illustration by Salma Price-Nell at thesalsacreative.com
Design by Blok Graphic

British Library Cataloguing-in-Publication Data
A catalogue record for this book is available from the British Library

Printed in the EU by Hussar

This book has been printed on paper that is sourced and harvested
from sustainable forests and is FSC accredited

Pinter & Martin Ltd
6 Effra Parade
London SW2 1PS

pinterandmartin.com

To my lovely little family
To all the amazing, strong women

Contents

How to use this book

→ A very warm 'hello' and welcome to you!

This book has been written for pregnant women and their birth partners. The guidelines discussed are UK-based and are just that – guidelines. In the UK, maternity units' guidelines vary from Trust to Trust, and policies and guidelines are often changed and amended. Your midwife or obstetrician will be able to point you to the latest policies for your particular Trust.

It is always fantastic when a woman and her birth partner can join a local, in-person antenatal course and have the luxury of time and the opportunity to discuss topics with others, but not everyone has the time, money, ability or a local antenatal course available to do this. The aim of this book is to walk you through all the labour and birth topics typically covered in a traditional face-to-face course. It also acts as an easy recap and reminder for those who have been able to attend a course, or as a refresher if you are becoming a parent for a second time (or a third or more!).

You will also learn about hypnobirthing and how the mind and body can work together to help to create a positive birth experience. There are easy-to-follow, practical and useful hypnobirthing techniques for you to use during pregnancy, labour and beyond. All the hypnobirthing scripts that appear at the back of this book can be downloaded as MP3s.

The book is split into eight easy-to-follow sections, designed to mimic an eight-week antenatal course that covers hypnobirthing, labour and birth. You can read it section-by-section over a number of weeks, giving yourself chance to think about what you've learned, and make decisions about your pregnancy and birth, or you can read it more quickly if you are pushed for time or are looking for a recap. However you do it, I highly recommended that you read the whole book, even if you don't think all the chapters may apply to you, as it will help to prepare you for whatever happens on the day of the birth, and give you confidence that you have explored all the ideas and options that are discussed.

The eight sessions will give you a good general overview of your choices and options for labour and birth. They are a starting point for thinking about what you might like for your baby's birth and there is an invitation at the end of each chapter for you to read more widely about topics, with links to help you get started. Alongside discussions with your caregivers, I encourage you to carry out your own research, so you can make your own empowering and informed decisions.

I wish you all the very best on your amazing journey!

Introduction

In my capacity as an antenatal and hypnobirthing practitioner, I often meet expectant parents who are unaware they have choices. All too often I hear 'Am I allowed...?', or 'I was told I had to...', or 'They won't let me...' You absolutely do have options and choices, and the decision to accept or not accept something always lies with you – but this doesn't have to feel overwhelming.

Sometimes in birth there are decisions to be made. I have written this guide as a simple introduction to the possible decisions, choices and options you may have during your baby's birth, to use alongside guidance from your caregivers, including questions which may be helpful to ask. I hope that it will help you as you prepare for the birth of your baby.

Having a baby and becoming a mother or a father is, of course, a life-changing experience. The circumstances of the birth, and how you and your partner feel as it all unfolds, can have long-lasting effects: ask any parent about their memories of their children's births and you will usually find that they remember it all in great detail, whether positive or negative.

My hope is that reading this book, and thinking about your choices, will help to ensure that you embark on parenthood feeling supported and informed, and able to ask questions of those who are caring for you.

Informed decision-making

I mention this here because it underpins much of what we will discuss later on. For your consent (to procedures, or to interventions) to be valid it must be voluntary and informed. Your legal right to informed consent means that your healthcare provider is responsible for explaining:

- Why this type of care is being offered
- What it would involve
- The harms and benefits that are associated with this type of care
- Alternatives to this care, and the harms and benefits of those other options
- The possibility of doing nothing at the present time

Informed consent is about having discussions with your midwife or doctor to help you to decide and agree on what will and will not be done to your body and how these decisions may affect you and your baby. If time allows, you can say 'Please show me the best conducted research on the evidence for 'X' for my specific situation so I can make an informed decision'.

Despite there being a common set of NICE (National Institute for Health & Care Excellence) guidelines for care during late pregnancy and labour, not all hospitals operate the same way and, at times, what may be suggested or recommended could just be the opinion of your midwife/doctor. You are entitled to ask for a second opinion if you are not in agreement or are unsure about anything.

Sometimes, during the course of pregnancy or labour an unexpected complication may arise and your midwife may suggest a way to proceed. Your midwife may ask how you feel about 'X, Y or Z' and it can be hard to know how best to go forward. It is absolutely fine to let the midwife know what your preferences are, and providing it is not an emergency situation (and it will be obvious if it is), you can ask as many questions as you want to. Asking questions can help you to gather information, feel involved and make informed decisions, rather than making decisions based around fear and the unknown, or feeling pushed into a decision without fully understanding it.

Different midwives have different approaches and, as wonderful as midwives are, they are only human and, like the rest of us, may have a preferred way of doing something – but there may be another way of achieving the same result, whatever it may be. It is always worthwhile asking questions. Gathering information and advocating for you can be a big part of a birth partner's role. In labour he or she can then relay any information back to you so you can be involved in any decision-making during the birth itself. For some suggestions for questions you could ask, and an outline of the BRAIN tool for making decisions, see page 57.

Informed decision-making makes for a positive birth. If you and your partner feel that you are able to ask relevant questions, gather information and understand things fully before agreeing to something, you will more likely feel empowered. This is so important. Asking a few questions and feeling respected and listened to can potentially change the course of your whole birth experience.

Of course, some women choose not to ask any questions and are happy to go with whatever suggestions are being made without discussion, and this too is a valid choice if that feels right for them.

"

Let's talk about the stages of labour

"

In the first session we talk about:

- The different parts of labour and birth and how your partner can help you along the way, starting with early labour: is this the real deal and have things finally started?

- How might labour surges feel?

- How to know when you are in active labour and whether or not it's time to start to think about going in, or time to update your midwife if you're planning a homebirth.

- We'll cover the journey in and your options around delivering the placenta. We'll also take a look at some signs that mean you should definitely get in touch with the labour ward, or go straight in.

Chapter one

The first two stages of labour and what to expect

→ Throughout this book I use the word 'surges' instead of 'contractions' – this is just a different and perhaps more positive word to describe the work of the uterus. You will likely hear both terms used during your pregnancy and labour.

The labour I describe below is a 'textbook' labour – many labours do not follow this clearly defined, textbook path as all women labour in their own individual way, each with a different pattern and length of the so-called stages.

You will hear of labour being divided into three stages – but this may be more for record-keeping than anything else. However, as you will hear the three stages mentioned during your pregnancy and labour, in this chapter we go through each one in turn.

You have probably heard of dilation of the cervix, or the cervix needing to open from 0cm to 10cm. The cervix is found internally – it is at the top of the vagina/birth canal and is the opening to the uterus/ the neck of the womb. During pregnancy, a woman's cervix is normally closed and has a mucous plug in it to keep out infection, which is called a 'show' when it comes away. Before dilation starts the cervix is around 3cm long, firm and points slightly towards your back.

1. The cervix is thick, long and firm. In preparation for the start of labour the cervix first needs to move from a posterior position (pointing towards your back) to an anterior position, so it is pointing more towards the front. Then it needs to shorten and soften, which is sometimes referred to as 'ripening'.

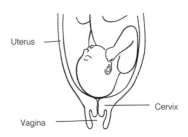

Uterus

Cervix

Vagina

Not effaced, not dilated

This ripening can start in late pregnancy before labour begins, or in early labour. Some women notice the mucous plug coming away (known as a 'show'). The mucous-like discharge is mixed with blood so it is usually pinky or a bit bloody. This is not always a sign that labour is imminent, but it is a sign that the body is getting ready and the cervix is starting to soften and open.

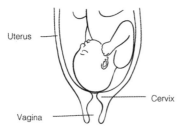

Uterus

Cervix

Vagina

Fully effaced, 2cm dilated

2. As you can see, the cervix in image 2 is fully effaced (thinned out) and has started to open (dilate). This is what your surges do – the strong muscular work of the surges draws the cervix up into the body of the uterus and it becomes thinner and then opens.

3. This shows a fully dilated cervix. As the cervix is internal, at the top of the vagina, you will not know how dilated you are unless you examine yourself or a midwife does this for you. Sometimes women know instinctively how far along in their labour they are, and a midwife can often tell by closely observing a woman's behaviour. If women have practised hypnobirthing, they can often appear

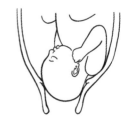

Fully effaced, fully dilated to 10cm

very calm late on in their labours, which may mean that those caring for them underestimate how far their labour has progressed. Therefore, it is important to tell your midwife if you are using hypnobirthing techniques.

Signs that your body is getting ready for labour (pre-labour)

- Increased practice surges, or Braxton Hicks contractions. Many women find these painless and are sometimes unaware they are having them, or they may notice their bump go hard and tight for a short while. Other women feel them strongly or get a period cramp-type sensation. Sometimes women have runs of Braxton Hicks for several days before the process of labour starts.
- Backache, or a pre-menstrual feeling.
- Waters releasing – this can be a gush, sometimes with an audible 'pop', or it can be a trickle. It can occur before labour starts or during it. You should let your maternity unit know when your waters have released.
- A show – the mucous plug can sometimes come away.
- The start of surges.
- Feeling different: maybe feeling restless, irritable or not sleeping well.
- An upset stomach, diarrhoea or a frequent need to open your bowels. This is caused by changes in the levels of certain hormones your body releases before labour starts. Don't worry about this, it is positive: the body is making as much room as possible for your baby's journey out.
- Nesting instinct – an urge to get your home in order and everything ready.
- 'Lightening' – this is the term used to describe the baby's head moving into your pelvis. Women usually feel that they can breathe more easily after this, as when the baby 'drops' there is more room for your lungs. This often happens a few weeks before labour starts.

As there can be an overlap between pre-labour and the start of labour itself, you may initially find it hard to tell whether or not labour has really started.

What do surges feel like?

This varies from woman to woman. Some women feel them very strongly and others just feel a tightening sensation.

Surges can be felt in the groin, lower abdomen and sometimes down the tops of the legs. Some women feel uncomfortable around their bump and back or experience a heavy feeling low down in their pelvis. Often surges start off short and mild, with long gaps in between each one, and as labour progresses the surges get longer, stronger and closer together. Some women experience regular, strong surges right from the start.

When labour starts – the first stage

The first stage of labour includes 'early/pre-labour' and 'active labour', sometimes called 'established labour'. As a rough guide, early labour is when surges are opening the cervix from 0–4cm, and the active stage of labour is when the cervix is opening from 4–10cm.

Early labour

During this stage surges are usually (though not always) irregular, perhaps coming every 15–20 minutes and lasting around 20–30 seconds. They may peter out, then start up again.

Labour can start at any time of the day or night. It often starts at night when you feel safe and secure and it is dark, cosy and warm in bed. Your brain and body think 'Ah, this is a good, safe time and place to go into labour!' As exciting as it is, resist waking your partner if it's the middle of the night, and instead try to go back to sleep, or at least rest with your phone turned off so you're not distracted by it. Your body will be grateful for the rest both now and later on. Putting on one of the hypnobirthing MP3s may help you to relax or even sleep for a while. If you wake your partner up they may leap into action and their excited energy will prevent you from being able to doze off again.

How can you help yourself in early labour?

- Have a warm bath (not too hot).
- Eat! Go with what you fancy, but high-fat foods may make you feel sick and your digestive system needs to rest. Not eating in labour can lead to feeling tired and weak later on, which can lead to unnecessary interventions. You could try toast, cereal, pasta, soup or sandwiches. Stay hydrated too.
- If you like cooking, distractions such as baking a cake or making a dish you haven't done before are useful, as you're focused on the recipe, you're upright and moving around which helps labour along, and you'll have a lovely meal or cake to enjoy at the end, or to come back to once your baby has arrived. Remember, surges are usually

mild in early labour, so it's quite possible you could manage to do this if it's of interest.

- Go for a local, relaxing walk.
- Use a birth ball.
- Rest with a book.
- Try to sleep.
- Use a hot water bottle wherever it's needed.
- Watch or listen to comedy or a light-hearted box set – not only is this distracting, but laughter is also relaxing and produces feel-good hormones such as oxytocin and endorphins, which help keep labour progressing beautifully.
- If you are using a TENS machine, the best time to put it on is in early labour. (A TENS machine is a form of pain management which we cover later – see page 156).

The first stage of labour is usually the longest, but of course this varies hugely from woman to woman. For first-time mothers it can be anything from eight hours to 18+ hours, with subsequent births often being quicker. The hormones released during labour distort your perception of time, so labour doesn't always necessarily feel as long as it is.

Staying at home during the first stage has many benefits, one of which is that a familiar and relaxing environment helps labour progress smoothly. At home you can get into your own space/zone more easily as it's your territory and you have all your home comforts around you. You can eat and drink what and when you like, rest in your own bed and come and go as you please.

If you want to, you can call the labour ward during this stage to seek reassurance from a midwife who will be happy to answer any questions you have.

Active labour (also called 'established labour')

In active labour typically your surges become longer, stronger, closer together and of increased intensity, each one requiring all your attention and focus. As a rough guide, at the start of active labour surges will be coming around every 3–4 minutes and last about a minute, and will have been doing this for at least an hour. But do remember that we are talking about a textbook labour! All women experience labour differently, with some starting off with regular, strong surges and others never getting into a regular pattern. It's far better to listen to your body and how you feel rather than getting too caught up in numbers and timings.

Tune into your body and how you are feeling. If you no longer want to chat through your surges, but instead want to stop what you're doing, turn your focus inwards and use deep breathing to help you, then you are probably in active labour. When your partner notices this change in you he or she can discreetly start to time your surges – when you call the labour ward to say you want to come in they will ask how frequently the surges have been coming and for how long.

You may feel hot and may not be interested in eating or talking much. You may also start to feel less inhibited, which is great as you are then able to follow your body's lead.

The intensity of the surges encourages you to move and get into one or many of the positions you will have practised during your pregnancy (more on positions for labour later, see Chapter 10). Following your body's lead and moving, rocking and swaying makes labour feel more manageable and helps your baby get into a good position, as well as increasing the release of some of the fantastic birthing hormones.

If you are planning a birth in hospital or at a birth centre (see Chapter 5), then this is the time to get ready to go in. If you are planning a home birth, let your home birth midwife know that you feel you are in active labour.

When you call to say you feel that you are in active labour and would like to come in to the labour ward or birth centre, the midwife may want to speak with you during several surges as part of the assessment to try to gauge how you are responding to them. She will also want to get a bit of background information from your partner.

As mentioned before, if you have prepared using hypnobirthing always let the midwife know, as you will likely appear calmer than expected for a woman in active labour. Trust your body and what you are feeling rather than how you are expected to be behaving.

Transition
Transition is the last part of the first stage of labour, when you move into the second stage. Waters may release at this stage, or just before it. A lot of women find this stage particularly challenging as the surges are usually very intense and it feels like they are back-to-back with barely

any gap in between them. It's the shortest part of the labour. Often women experience a big moment of self-doubt at this stage and you may feel the urge to push. You may also feel a bit shaky or sick – this is due to raised adrenalin levels. Raised adrenalin will give you the energy to soon start to push your baby out, but it also takes you out of the zone you were in and you suddenly take stock, perhaps saying 'How much longer?' or 'I've had enough of this now, I've changed my mind. I'll have this baby tomorrow!' You may become a bit irate and fed up with it all, or go deeper into yourself. This is all really normal, and it's not a sign that anything is wrong. You are so close now!

How can you help yourself during active labour?

If you have not already started to focus on your breathing, now is the time. Slow, deep, calming breathing, with the out-breath a little longer than the in-breath, will help to keep you relaxed and focused as you leave home to transfer into hospital, or while you wait for your home birth midwife to arrive.

- Slow, deep, calm breathing will save energy and bring you and your baby increased oxygen, helping your uterus to do its incredible job.
- Massage from your birth partner may be beneficial, though some women prefer not to be touched during active labour.
- Stay hydrated and eat what you fancy.
- Change position and use a birth ball.
- Try a birth pool if it's available, or have a shower.
- Use a hot water bottle.
- Empty your bladder regularly.

Your birth partner can remind you to do all of these things.

How can you help yourself during transition?

It's hard to know when you are in the midst of labour that you are in transition. If your partner notices a change in your behaviour he or she could ask the midwife out of earshot and if they think you are in transition, they can give you lots of reassurance that you are very close now. Co-breathing (where your partner breathes along with you) may be of help.

Take one surge at a time and continue breathing deeply until you reach the end of transition. If you haven't yet felt the urge to push, you will usually feel pressure in the back passage, which is followed by an urge to bear down or push. This is the start of the second stage of labour, or the 'pushing' or 'breathing down' stage.

There is usually a lull in surges before the second stage starts and you can rest a little.

The second stage of labour

The second stage of labour starts when the cervix has fully dilated and ends when the baby is born. It can be very short, or as long as 2-3 hours for a first-time mother.

The start of the second stage of labour is the journey the baby takes through the vagina (or some call it the birth canal) to the outside world. Surges are usually intense and expulsive, lasting about 1-1½ minutes as your powerful uterus nudges your baby down and out of your vagina. Many liken it to the sensation of needing to open the bowels.

Breathing and positions for the second stage

There is more later in the book on breathing techniques, but during surges it is important to continue deep breathing, bringing valuable oxygen to your baby and uterus. Rather than holding your breath and pushing hard against your body, work with your body and follow its lead. It knows what it is doing.

It may help to take a deep breath in through your nose (or mouth if you have a blocked nose) and then, with your jaw relaxed, breathe out firmly but gently, sending the breath out through your nose and down the back of your throat, down towards your pelvic floor, giving your baby a helpful nudge downwards when the urge to push is felt. You can practise this type of breathing when you are on the toilet and need to open your bowels - you'll see how useful it is!

There is nothing wrong with pushing if you are working with your body rather than coached pushing where someone tells you how and when to push. (More on this later.)

You may want to repeat this breathing technique 3-4 times during the longer, expulsive second-stage surges. Each oxygen-fuelled, powerful breath will help your baby on their journey down.

Move around and change position as your body dictates. You may like to try not to lie flat, or semi-flat (you can read more about useful labour and birth positions later in the book). Remember to empty your bladder regularly, particularly if your breathing down/pushing efforts are ineffective.

How you can help yourself during second stage

- Maintain long, deep, powerful breaths, which focus downwards, helping your baby on their journey into the world.
- Consider which positions you can adopt that will create room in your pelvis.
- If you are concerned about opening your bowels at this stage, you can sit on the toilet or straddle the toilet back to front, leaning over on the cistern (put a pillow on it) – this is safe to do and a great position to be in both now and early on in your labour. The toilet is a place we go to when we want to feel private and when we want our body to open up and release.
- Having sips of coconut water or another healthy alternative, to replace lost electrolytes, can help boost energy. It's important to keep hydrated throughout your labour.
- Again, remember to empty your bladder regularly.
- Know that each powerful surge is bringing you closer to finally meeting your baby!

Vaginal examinations

Examinations are offered on arrival at hospital, or when your home birth midwife arrives, to check if you are in active labour. Once you are in active labour they are usually offered at around four-hourly intervals, as part of assessing your progress, among other things. Your consent should always be given before any intervention takes place. If you wish, you can request an examination.

Sometimes you may choose not to have any examinations. Women may find them invasive and uncomfortable, or have other personal reasons for not wanting them. Some women prefer not to know how many centimetres they are dilated and instead be guided by their own bodies, or would rather not be given a number, but simply be told whether things are progressing well. Let your midwife know your preferences.

You can choose to accept one initial vaginal examination and then decline any others, or you can agree to have examinations as offered. It is always your choice whether you consent to an examination or not. You do not necessarily have to be lying flat on the bed to have one; for example you could be in an all-fours position or in a birth pool.

Examinations offer a 'screen shot' of a moment, and knowing the dilation of the cervix does not predict when a woman will give birth. Some women can progress very quickly if the environment is right and they feel safe and secure. Conversely, if a woman becomes anxious or unable to relax her labour may slow down and she may pause at, for example, 6cm, if in her mind she is unable to let go, or there are other factors in play such as the position of the baby.

Sometimes a midwife may inadvertently break the waters during an examination. Waters are the amniotic fluid that surrounds the baby. The waters act as a cushion between the baby's head and the cervix, and when they release this cushioning disappears, which can make surges feel more intense. This may change the path of labour if a woman now feels she needs some pain relief.

Once the waters have released, a 'clock' is started on progression of labour, meaning that if labour does not progress within certain parameters after this point, interventions will be offered to augment (speed up) the labour. These come with their own risks, which you can ask questions about before deciding to accept or decline. If you choose to decline interventions it's very important to keep an eye on your baby's movements. You may be given guidance from your midwife about regularly taking your own temperature every few hours, as a raised temperature could indicate an infection.

You can reflect on your feelings about examinations and interventions to speed up labour, and record your preferences in your birth plan (see Chapter 21).

Chapter two

The third stage – delivery of the placenta

→ This is the stage from when your baby is born until the placenta (sometimes called afterbirth) is birthed and any bleeding is under control. During the third stage the placenta starts to come away from the wall of the uterus and then it is moved down into the vagina by the surges, where it is birthed.

Keeping warm, having a dimly lit and private environment, holding your baby skin-to-skin and breastfeeding (if you're planning on doing this) can help with the third stage, as all of these things help with the production of the hormone oxytocin, aiding the safe delivery of the placenta.

There are two types of third stage and you can think about what you would prefer now, or at the time. How your birth has gone may impact your decision.

Active management

This is made up of three components. You are given an injection in the thigh that helps the uterus to contract strongly, the cord is clamped and cut 1-5 minutes after the injection and the midwife carefully guides the placenta out via the cord while supporting your uterus externally with her hand – this is called controlled cord traction. Active management shortens the third stage and reduces the risk of heavy blood loss. It increases the chance of nausea and vomiting.

Physiological management

This means there is no intervention. You hold your baby while they are still attached by the umbilical cord to the placenta.

During a physiological third stage the cord is not clamped and cut – either until it stops pulsating (this 'pulsating' is the baby's blood moving from the placenta and cord into the baby) or until the placenta is delivered. The baby gets their full quota of blood and the placenta is delivered by maternal effort. If you choose to have a physiological third stage and then you start to bleed more heavily than is usual, your midwife will be able to give you the injection as per the managed third stage. If everything has gone well with your labour and you don't have any risk factors for heavy bleeding a physiological third stage doesn't make it more likely that you'll bleed very heavily.

Why might you opt for a physiological third stage?

Around a third of the baby's blood is inside the cord and placenta at any one time. If the cord is clamped and cut straight away, this blood, which is rich in iron and stem cells, is not passed to its rightful owner – the baby.

By waiting for 10-20 minutes – or however long it takes before the cord goes white – before clamping and cutting the cord, the oxygenated blood from the placenta and cord will have passed into the baby. This means they will have good iron stores and enough blood to fill all the vessels around their lungs, making breathing easier. With this way of birthing the placenta the cord is usually clamped and cut after the placenta has been delivered, or when the cord has stopped pulsating and has turned white.

Why might you choose an actively managed third stage?

Sometimes it may be safer to have active management of the third stage. If there is heavy bleeding, or if the birth has been very long, complicated or medically managed – for example, if you have had your labour induced (when labour is started using drugs) or augmented (when labour is speeded up using drugs), or if you have had an assisted birth (using forceps or ventouse) – an active third stage is safer as the risk of heavy blood loss increases when things are less straightforward.

You can make a decision about how you want to have the third stage in advance and then see how the birth progresses. You could start off with a planned physiological third stage and then opt for the injection at any point, or you can choose active management.

It may also be possible to have optimal cord clamping at a caesarean birth, though this would need to be discussed in advance – or at the time of decision if it is an unplanned caesarean (an unplanned caesarean is when the decision is made to move to a caesarean birth during labour).

You can always change your mind about your choices and talk to your midwife about it at the time. If you do opt for a managed third stage, you can usually wait up to five minutes before the cord is clamped and cut, meaning your baby will receive the majority of their blood.

How can you help yourself during the third stage?

- Hold your baby skin-to-skin (their bare skin against your bare skin). There is some evidence that when women have skin-to-skin contact with their baby after birth and breastfeed them there are fewer postpartum haemorrhages (PPH).
- Breastfeed your baby if this is something you are planning to do, as this will help to release the placenta.
- Adopt an upright position to utilise gravity to help the placenta to come out – kneeling on the bed is a good position.
- Keep the lights low.
- Keep warm – some women are shivery after birth, due to increased

adrenalin. Increased adrenalin can slow the third stage down. Have your partner put a blanket around you.

- There is a saying: 'No hatting, no patting, no chatting' (coined by midwife Carla Hartley), meaning just that! It reflects the need for a quiet (no chatting) and calm environment after birth, leaving the mother to hold her baby (no patting) and breathe in their scent (no hatting). All this fosters high levels of oxytocin that are needed to complete the birth safely.
- Empty your bladder – a full bladder can slow the third stage down.

Chapter three

Stay at home or go in?

 You should call the labour ward or your home birth team if:

- You experience reduced movements. This is important throughout your pregnancy as well as during your labour. Movements should not lessen or slow down the bigger your baby gets – there will not be any 'somersaults' in the later weeks of pregnancy due to the lack of room, but the amount of movement you feel should be the same as before. Babies' movements do not slow down as a pregnancy progresses.
- You have any fluid loss, or you think your waters may have released. Waters should be clear – if they are tinged with brown or green, or have any strong odour, you should go in and get it checked out. It may mean your baby needs monitoring.
- You have any blood loss.
- You have a headache or visual disturbances such as colours, patches or blurred vision.
- You have sudden swelling of the face and hands.

- You have a rash, or itching.
- You are in any constant abdominal pain, especially in your upper abdomen, are experiencing nausea or have pain passing urine.
- You have a raised temperature or you just do not feel 'right'.
- You are feeling generally unwell or extremely fatigued.

If you have any concerns whatsoever, don't hesitate to call the labour ward. They are open 24/7 and they are there for you and you are not wasting their time by contacting them with your concerns. Don't be fobbed off if you feel something is not right. Call as many times as you need to and never put things off or wait to see how you or your baby are the following day.

Going in

It can sometimes be hard antenatally to understand how you will know when you are in labour and how you will know when to transfer in.

As discussed in Chapter 1, there may be a time when you are wondering 'Is this it, has my labour started for real?' You may wonder if you are just having more Braxton Hicks contractions.

Usually, it becomes obvious that you are in labour as surges get closer together, become longer and stronger and take all of your attention to manage. You no longer want to chat through them, but instead want to turn your focus inwards and breathe through them.

If things are ticking along and you are having a straightforward pregnancy, staying at home as long as possible has many benefits, including:

- It's your familiar environment, where you feel relaxed.
- You can eat and drink whatever you want; no need to get hot drinks from a machine.
- You can have a bath or shower in your own space.
- You can rest in your own familiar and comforting bed.
- You can watch a comedy box set or something that makes you relax and laugh while moving and bouncing on your birth ball – distractions are so useful.
- You have everything at home that you need and it is the best place to be for early labour.

- You're more likely to have a smoother labour with fewer interventions if you stay at home until you are in active labour.

Usually women want to transfer in or ask their home birth midwife to come over when surges have been coming every 3-4 minutes, lasting about a minute, for at least an hour. Typically, this is how surges will feel in active labour, though, to run the risk of repeating myself, we are of course all different and some women never get into a regular pattern of surges. Go with how you are feeling, rather than whether you've ticked the box of having 3-4 surges in a 10-minute period.

Still unsure? In the absence of a history of a precipitate (very fast) labour, if you find yourself wondering whether it's time to go in, or you are still chatting through surges, it is probably too early. It could be that just a short while later you turn to your partner and say 'I want to go in – now!', but any time before that you really are better off nesting at home. If this is your second or more pregnancy talk to your midwife about when it is best to head in to hospital or call her (if it's a home birth) as sometimes subsequent births can be quicker.

The journey in

It is quite common for labour to slow down or completely stall when a woman leaves her familiar home and goes into the relative unknown. As well as feeling excited, you may feel a little anxious, which is perfectly understandable.

Anxiety increases adrenalin levels in the body, which can hinder labour. We are the same as our mammal relatives – if a labouring animal notices a predator, feels anxious, or out of her safe place (home, for us humans), her adrenalin levels rise and pause her labour. She will attempt to find a safe place to hide until the threat goes away, and her labour will restart when she feels relaxed and safe. We are the same – but luckily we don't have any predators lurking.

To help with the transition from home to your chosen place of birth, if possible it is well worth doing a tour of the birth centre or hospital beforehand. Not all hospitals offer a tour, but many have an online version which will give you an idea of what the rooms are like.

It's also good to be familiar with the parking situation at your place of birth – get rid of as many 'unknowns' as you can in advance. Some hospitals have large car parks with sections dedicated to maternity.

Others are very tight for space, especially in London, and have parking restrictions at certain times of the day in the surrounding roads. Doing your homework first is helpful. You may also want to check out what parking app you need to have downloaded and ready with your bank card details already set up – and have plenty of change in the car as a back-up.

Many people choose to take a taxi instead, and of course not everyone has access to a car. If you are planning on taking a taxi ring around and find around three different cab companies that are willing to take a woman in labour, as not all do. Your local hospital may be able to recommend taxi companies that will take labouring women. You can explain that you will bring a towel to sit on (the usual concern is about waters leaking into their upholstery).

If you own a car, your partner can then get a cab home after the birth and come and pick you up in your own car, with your car seat fitted and ready to take your precious cargo home.

Another option is to draft in a family member or friend to be on call to take you to hospital.

How to help yourself when transferring from home

- Visit your chosen place of birth in advance.
- Assuming all has been well in your pregnancy, try not to be tempted to go in too early – wait until your surges are strong, long and close together.
- Try to stay in your 'zone' by blocking out external noise and light.
- Plug in your headphones and listen to music or your favourite hypnobirthing MP3. Or use earplugs to block out the world and keep your focus inwards.
- Put on an eye mask or sunglasses in the taxi.
- Cover up with a big hoody.
- Try your best to keep your senses turned inwards and ask your partner to deal with the admin and questions.
- Don't worry about how you look – you'll probably never see any of these people again.

Keep this going until you get into your labour or birth centre room, and then you can adjust the room as you see fit to make it cosy and dark.

End-of-session summary

You've now completed the first three chapters covering the stages of labour and thinking about when to go into hospital.

Before moving on, I invite you to do a little research of your own on the topics we've covered so far. This will help to consolidate your learning. Below are some links to get you started – see what else comes up on these topics when you have a search.

- NICE guidelines. NICE is an acronym for the National Institute for Health & Care Excellence. It is a great resource for information on the recommended guidelines for caring for women before, during and after birth. Start with the guideline on intrapartum care for healthy women and babies – intrapartum is the time period from the start of labour to the delivery of the placenta. It's clinical guideline CG190 and can be found here: **www.nice.org.uk/guidance/ cg190/resources/intrapartum-care-for-healthy-women-and-babies- pdf-35109866447557**
- Early signs that labour may have started **www.nct.org.uk/labour-birth/ your-guide-labour/early-signs-labour**
- Vaginal examinations in labour **www.aims.org.uk/information/item/ vaginal-examinations-in-labour**
- Third stage of labour **www.babycentre.co.uk/x1043341/what-is-delayed- cord-clamping-and-should-i-do-it?fbclid=IwAR37lG7ns8BOn2Hqehew03 BxqkjOoyrSJ_NvitZP_zrA3r2OpTcYbDqRZ6o**

"

Let's talk about your birth environment

"

In the second session we talk about:

- What helps and hinders labour and what you and your birth partner can do to maximise a straightforward birth.

- We'll take a look at place of birth – home birth, birth centre, labour ward. What support do you get at each one, what resources are available, what are the advantages and disadvantages of each place of birth and how does it all work?

- We'll also consider the birth partner's very important role and how best they can communicate with your healthcare providers, what questions would be useful to ask and how best he or she can support you during labour and birth. There's a birth partner's 'to-do list for labour' and an easy checklist to help you during the third stage (delivery of the placenta).

Chapter four

Hormones and environment – what helps and hinders labour?

→ When the long-awaited day finally comes around and you give birth to a tiny, brand new human being you will be at your most powerful. A woman in labour is an incredible force – but she is also vulnerable. Your senses will be heightened and how you are feeling and your immediate environment will have a huge impact on how well your labour progresses.

To help things go super smoothly, you need to feel safe, secure, warm and – most importantly – as undisturbed as is possible. Ideally you won't be 'watched over', or unduly interrupted or questioned. As birth is pretty primal, you want the neocortex – the 'newer' part of the brain, the rational, logical part which, among other things, is involved in conscious thought and reasoning – well and truly out of the picture so you can get into your own private zone.

Even small things such as someone entering the room or turning on a bright overhead light can bring you out of this zone. Your immediate environment plays such a big part in how your birth unfolds. Giving birth is the most private and personal thing you will ever do and you need to create a similar environment for birth as you have when getting intimate with your loved one. For most this would be an environment with low lighting, not having people wandering in and out, not having someone asking us how we are progressing and 'can we hurry up a bit', not having someone make suggestions on how we should be 'doing it' and not being told what position we should be in. Can you imagine this happening when you're getting intimate with your partner?! Nothing would be more likely to shut your body down, clamp it up and cause everything to stall, and the same applies for birth.

Think of when you have watched an animal give birth on a wildlife documentary. The mother will give birth when she feels safe, usually hidden away and in the dark. She will appear calm and relaxed and will use movement and low, quiet noises and sounds to help her. If she feels threatened, she will halt her labour until she feels safe again.

We fellow mammals need the same quiet, dark, private conditions to give birth well and feeling observed, fearful or anxious will have a very real effect on the progress of our labour. Interruptions, (usually) giving birth in a public building, bright lights, being poked and prodded by a relative stranger and potentially being told to 'hurry up or we'll need to intervene' are all a huge hindrance and take you out of your all-important private birthing zone. Without going into great detail about birthing hormones, I do want to explain them briefly and how they are affected by the immediate environment.

Oxytocin

Oxytocin is the powerhouse hormone of labour. We don't know exactly what starts labour, but oxytocin is one hormone that affects the length and strength of surges. Released in pulses, it helps the muscles of the uterus work to open the cervix. This muscular work signals the brain to produce more oxytocin, keeping labour beautifully effective and rhythmic. Oxytocin is also known as the 'hormone of love', because, among other things, it is released when couples make love (for women, breast/nipple stimulation and orgasm will release oxytocin), and when people feel relaxed, happy, safe and secure. A dark environment promotes the release of oxytocin (the hormone melatonin helps with that) and, coupled with high levels of endorphins, will help to make labour feel more comfortable and keep you feeling calm.

Adrenalin and noradrenalin

The fight-or-flight hormones, adrenalin and noradrenalin, are hormones produced by the body in response to stresses such as excitement, hunger, fear/anxiety and cold. When these hormones kick in, the body gets ready to 'freeze, fight or flight'. These hormones inhibit oxytocin release.

It is normal for there to be adrenalin present during the transition part of labour (towards the end of the first stage) and when the uterus is nudging the baby out. However, if you have high levels of adrenalin during your whole labour, this can interfere with your surges, slowing or even stopping labour. Blood flow to the uterus and placenta is reduced, which not only affects labour and comfort levels, but can also affect the baby.

'Fight or flight' is the perfect response for emergency life-or-death situations, and for wild animals giving birth this reflex inhibits labour and sends blood to the major muscle groups, so the birthing mother can choose to flee from a threat or give birth quickly. We are lucky enough not to have such threats when we give birth – birth is generally very safe – but as already mentioned, bright lights, feeling observed, frequent interruptions and feeling fearful and anxious can quite easily tip a woman into this state. As a result, surges are likely to be less efficient and more painful, and labour may slow or even stop completely.

Beta-endorphins

These are naturally occurring opiates, which are our very own, in-house, powerful painkillers, with similar properties to morphine and pethidine. Released whenever there is physical activity and when the body is working hard, in labour they will help reduce pain and help you feel calm and 'zoned out'. Interruptions and chatter inhibit their production, so keep this to a minimum to allow yourself to get into a quiet, private 'labour land' rhythm. This is a big part of the birth partner's role: they can help to protect your environment.

What will help you feel safe, secure and uninhibited?

- **Lights out/lights low.** Melatonin is a hormone that helps us sleep and its production peaks when it is dark. Melatonin helps with the release of oxytocin so keeping things as dark as possible will help with this process. If you are planning a home birth you will have more control over lighting, but you can still achieve this in a birth centre or labour ward as they both usually have dimmer switches and blinds. You could also bring in portable blackout blinds along with battery-operated candles or fairy lights for gentle, soft lighting. You can also bring in an eye mask or even sunglasses to shut out the outside world. The room is yours to make your own.

- **Touch (if wanted!)**. Hugging, kissing, cuddling, stroking/massage: loving touch helps to release oxytocin and endorphins and it's a way of communicating without speaking. A long hug from your partner or birth partner will make you feel safe; his or her familiar scent and touch will help to settle and calm you.

- **Movement.** Try rocking, swaying, using a birth ball, using the lowered bed as a prop to lean on rather than lie on, making a figure of eight with your hips, getting on all fours and leaning back and forth, sitting on the toilet, leaning forward onto a wall or raising the bed so you can stand up and lean onto it while resting on pillows... follow your body's lead. Movement helps the baby get into a good position and makes things feel more manageable for you. It also means there will be good blood flow to the placenta and uterus, helping the baby, and may even shave some time off your labour.

- **Quiet.** This is not saying you cannot interact with or talk to anyone, but keeping interruptions to a minimum, and avoiding complex questions that take you out of your zone and stimulate your neocortex, is helpful. Birth can of course be noisy, and making sounds can be releasing and this should not be restricted. But make sure that your birth partner ensures the environment you are in lends itself to letting you release, relax and go into yourself. Think of other mammals and how and where they give birth. Each interrupted surge is one that is less efficient. Make each incredible, amazing and powerful surge count.

- **Senses.** Smell is one of the most powerful. The familiar smell of home, whether on a blanket, pillow or pyjamas, or a scent that you like on a piece of fabric, such as a few drops of lavender oil, can increase comfort levels. If you've practiced using hypnobirthing use the same anchor scent you used when doing your practice.

- **Sounds.** Play one of the MP3s of the hypnobirthing scripts that are in this book that you have been listening to – its familiarity and the calming background music will ground you. You can also get a music playlist together or bring in ear plugs to block out the outside world.

- **Let go of fears** and trust that your body knows how to birth your baby. There are practical tools on how to start working on this later in the book.
- **Birth partners.** Your input is so important! Ensure the birth preferences document is read (yes, they are flexible, but they are your hopes and wishes and it is important that they are read). Ensure your partner has access to food and drink. Control the environment; keep unnecessary chatter at bay and protect your partner's space. Know that moments of self-doubt are usual for a woman in labour, particularly during transition, and speak to the midwife out of earshot if you feel concerned by this. If you're unsure what to do, just think 'Am I/is this helping to make her feel safe, secure and private?'

When you have an undisturbed birth, your hormones flow perfectly, increasing your safety and that of your baby. Interference with this hormonal flow can make birth more difficult and painful. Of course, there are things we cannot control during birth. However, there is also a lot we can do to help ensure that it unfolds as comfortably and smoothly as possible.

Chapter five

Deciding where to have your baby

→ At some point fairly early on in your pregnancy your midwife should talk to you about your options for where you would like to give birth to your baby. If this has not happened, you can ask to go through it at your next appointment.

You can give birth at home, or in a midwife-led unit (otherwise known as a 'birth centre', or 'home from home') or in the main delivery suite/labour ward. Midwife-led units may be either freestanding (not attached to a hospital – though there are not currently many of these in the UK) or alongside (in the same building as the main labour ward – this is more usual).

It is well worth doing some research into each of the options discussed below, and if you have more than one hospital near you, look at each one and do a tour of each if it is available.

If you have several hospitals in your area you can choose which one you want to give birth in. Usually you can self-refer online – talk to your midwife or call the hospital's maternity phone number if you're unsure how to do this. Bear in mind that if you are planning a home birth it is usual for the home birth team only to work with women within their catchment area. If your postcode is out of the catchment area for your chosen hospital it's always worth asking a senior midwife or the home birth team if they would consider caring for you – you'll never know unless you ask! Perhaps instead of saying 'I'm going to have a home birth' you could say to yourself 'I'm going to labour at home and see how I go – no pressure'.

Home birth

Some women like the idea of giving birth at home – a place where they are in control, they feel less like a patient, they are able to have a bath, and they can eat and drink whatever and whenever they want. It is easier to distract yourself at home and carry on as normal for longer. You can book a home birth with your midwife. When you go into labour you call your midwife and she or a member of her team, who you likely will already know or have met, will come out to you at home. When the birth is imminent, she will usually call a second midwife to help her. If you book a home birth you can change your mind at any time during your pregnancy – even during labour – and instead opt to go to the birth centre or labour ward.

What are the benefits of a home birth?

- If you plan a home birth you are more likely to have met the midwife who will take care of you during your labour in advance (if your home birth team offer what is called 'case loading', where a named midwife will provide continuity of care). This can help you feel more comfortable and relaxed. Research has shown that, understandably, labour usually progresses well at home when a woman knows her midwife.
- You are in your own domain, free to move around from room to room as you wish and eat and drink whatever you like, whenever you like.
- If you need to transfer into hospital, your midwife will go with you. She may stay if this is possible, or she may hand you over to the care of the hospital midwives on duty.
- There is less pressure to labour within a particular timeframe, which

means that fewer interventions are offered to speed up your labour.

- Should you require medical intervention your midwife will arrange for you to go to your local hospital.
- There is less chance of infection at a home birth.
- You really do get one-to-one care, as the midwife will be focusing on you and your baby and no one else. She will be regularly listening in to your baby's heartbeat and will not hesitate to suggest you transfer in if she suspects there is a problem – something she will do long before any situation becomes an emergency.
- Home birth is associated with improved breastfeeding outcomes.
- Midwives are highly skilled and trained, attending regular updates to refresh their skills on how to deal with emergencies.

The Birthplace study showed that for healthy women with straightforward pregnancies that are having a second or subsequent baby, home births are safe for the baby and may offer the following benefits:

- A lower chance of needing a caesarean birth
- A lower chance of needing an assisted delivery, i.e. forceps or ventouse
- Postpartum haemorrhage (excessive blood loss after having your baby) is significantly less likely after a home birth than after a hospital birth.

Home birth and safety

Medical emergencies can occur anywhere, regardless of where a woman gives birth – but do remember that giving birth is generally very safe.

As already mentioned, midwives are highly skilled and are trained to deal with any urgent situations while calling for further help. For example, if a postpartum haemorrhage were to occur, the midwife would have the initial drugs necessary, along with specific techniques to manage this, and would arrange a speedy transfer into hospital.

In some cases, a woman requesting a home birth may be encouraged to give birth in hospital, for example in the event of a pregnancy lasting longer than 42 weeks, or the baby being in a breech position. Some women with less straightforward pregnancies or less usual factors to consider choose to research the pros and cons of their specific situation and make an informed decision to still give birth at home.

What's available at a home birth?

- You can have a water birth at home if you hire a pool – in fact having a home birth is the only way to guarantee having a water birth, as the pool is there just for you. Sometimes you can find second-hand pools online, and just buy a new liner. Your home birth team may have a pool you can borrow.
- You can hire or buy a TENS machine and use this.
- You will have access to Entonox (gas and air).
- You may have access to either pethidine or diamorphine (opiates).

NICE guidance states that you should be supported and informed about your birthplace options. Your GP or midwife should not try to dissuade you from your choice unless they feel there is a genuine medical reason to do so. If there is a medical reason as to why something is being suggested then of course you'd be wise to discuss this and, if you want to, you can ask for sources of research and information on it so you can read up on it for yourself. But the decision is always yours and you are free to make your own choices even if your caregivers do not agree with you.

Birth centre

Sometimes a birth centre is referred to as a 'home from home' or a 'midwife-led suite'. Giving birth in a birth centre can be a great option for many women who have had straightforward pregnancies and is the 'default setting' for these women. Birth centres are run by midwives and do not routinely use medical interventions if labour is progressing well. As many labours do progress well, birth centres are a good alternative to giving birth on the labour ward.

Should you require any medical intervention you can transfer to the labour ward. Most birth centres are in the same building, and some are even on the same floor as the main hospital/labour ward, which many women find reassuring.

Advantages of using a birth centre

- Birth centres feel more homely and less clinical, which in turn can make you feel more relaxed.
- They are often more spacious, with more equipment available, such

as birthing stools, a sofa, mats, birth balls and padded floors or mats to comfortably kneel on.

- They may have a double bed available for after the birth for your birth partner to stay overnight, but this is sometimes tucked out of the way or folded up against the wall to encourage women not to hop up on it! This is because research shows that being upright and mobile during active labour has many benefits, including making labour feel more manageable and potentially shortening the second stage of labour.
- Within birth centres birth is seen as a normal event and having a straightforward birth is much more likely. Straightforward birth means giving birth vaginally, without any procedures or interventions such as assisted birth (forceps or ventouse), induction of labour or caesarean birth.
- Some birth centres allow you to stay in the room, with your partner and baby, for your whole stay, though you will need to transfer out and into the postnatal ward if someone wants to use the room. Usually you will transfer to the postnatal ward 1-2 hours or so after the birth.
- The midwives who work in a birth centre have often chosen this environment as they have a passionate interest in supporting women to birth with little or no intervention.
- You are less likely to have a serious PPH (postpartum haemorrhage) if you plan to give birth at home or in a midwife-led unit.

Disadvantages of using a birth centre

- If you decide you want an epidural or you or your baby require more careful monitoring then you'll need to leave the birth centre and transfer to the labour ward. If your birth centre is not located within the hospital, ask your midwife which unit you would transfer to and how long this would take.
- A room may not be available within the birth centre. If this is the case your birth partner can regularly ask if one has become available yet.

What's available at a birth centre?

- A water birth if there is a pool plumbed in or an inflatable one available. Pools may not be available in all rooms.
- You can hire or buy a TENS machine and use this.
- You will have access to Entonox (gas and air).

- Sometimes the midwives are trained in and can offer aromatherapy massage or reflexology.
- You will be able to adjust the lighting.
- Often you will be able to have pethidine or diamorphine for pain relief during labour should you want this.
- There is less equipment visible, which helps to give a feel of birth being a normal event.
- While the transfer may not happen instantly unless it is an emergency, you can always change your mind and transfer out of the birth centre and onto the labour ward should you wish to – for example if you decide you want an epidural (epidurals are not available in the birth centre).
- If your baby needs special care they will be transferred to the special care baby unit, which in most cases will be in the same building.

Hospital birth/labour ward

Some women choose to give birth on the labour ward as they find it reassuring or they are keen on having an epidural.

If you have had a less straightforward pregnancy and you are having consultant-led care, you will likely be offered the labour ward rather than the birth centre – though do say that you'd like to use the birth centre if this is something you're hoping for as this may be negotiable.

Being in the hospital environment makes it more likely that you will be offered interventions, which is something to bear in mind. There is also less privacy in a hospital setting.

Your care will still be provided by midwives, but doctors will be available if required. It is unlikely that you will have met your midwife in advance of your birth.

What is available on the labour ward?

- You will have access to an epidural, pethidine/diamorphine and Entonox (gas and air). You can bring a TENS machine in if you want to try this.
- Some labour wards have birthing pools available – ask your midwife or check your hospital's maternity website.
- Continuous electronic foetal monitoring for the baby, should this be required. Also additional monitoring of the mother.

Some women like to start in the birth centre and transfer to the labour ward if they feel they would like an epidural.

Once you are in your room on the labour ward you can make it your own. You may like to:

- Adjust the room e.g. dim the lights, close the blinds as discussed in the previous chapter.
- Cover any unused equipment with a scarf or blanket/towel to make it feel less clinical.
- Use a birth ball – this should be provided but you can bring your own.
- Raise or lower the bed so you are not tempted to get on it and therefore not move around much.
- Bring your playlist with a mini speaker.
- Bring an essential oil of your choice to breathe in from a piece of fabric or cotton wool ball.
- Cover the clock so you are not focused on it.

It is your choice whether you give birth at home or within a hospital, though of course it's important to discuss any pros and cons with your caregivers. Take time to research all the options and choose wherever you think you will feel most relaxed and safe.

You can always change your mind at any point, but if a home birth is something you are interested in you should make sure your midwives know this – the earlier the better.

If you feel you are not being supported in your choices by your midwife or consultant you can contact a senior midwife, consultant midwife or professional maternity advocate (PMA) by ringing your hospital or writing to/emailing him/her. Part of their role is to advocate for you and to work with you as best as they can to help you achieve the birth you are hoping for.

Chapter six

The birth partner's role

→ The role of the birth partner is so important. Sadly, it is not always possible to get continuous one-to-one support from our amazing but over-stretched midwives, so having the constant support of a familiar person is invaluable.

Birth partners can be the baby's father, dads, mums, partners, sisters, friends or a doula (more on doulas later). Usually a maximum of two supporters are allowed in the labour room or birth centre, although if you have a home birth you can have as many as you like. Remember though that the fewer interruptions a labouring woman has the better, so think about how you might feel giving birth in a room full of people, however lovely they are! As you already know, feeling observed can hinder labour, so it might be wise to keep birth partners to a minimum, though the choice is of course all yours.

A quick guide for birth partners

Read up on labour and birth – starting with this guide. Knowledge is power and you need to be on board and understand the decisions and choices your partner will potentially be faced with during labour and birth.

If possible, attend as many classes as you can – NHS ones are free and they also often run breastfeeding workshops, which you can attend together. The National Childbirth Trust (NCT) offers paid-for classes and some couples/women may be able to access classes at a subsidised cost. You can find out more at www.nct.org.uk.

Get organised and think ahead in terms of how you will get to the hospital or birth centre. Will you drive? If yes, keep the car well fuelled as you never know when it might be needed. Or are you going to take a cab or draft in a friend or family member? If driving, have money ready for parking or set up the relevant parking app on your phone in advance. There are also websites where you can organise hiring someone's unused driveway which is situated close to the hospital – this is often cheaper than paying for meters, but would only be useful if you knew when you had to be in hospital, for example for a scan appointment or a planned induction.

Pack the hospital bag together so you both know where and what everything is.

Draw up a birth plan/preferences together

While it is valuable to plan, visualise and affirm your ideal birth, planning for all eventualities is useful as birth can be unpredictable at times. Once you have jotted down your wishes for a straightforward birth, induction of labour and caesarean birth, put any 'what ifs' to one side and both go all out on focusing and visualising the birth you both want, doing any research which might help around this. There is a birth preferences template in this book, or you can follow the NHS one or a template your midwife may give you.

Massage

The power of loving touch can be comforting and is a lovely way of saying you are there for your partner without needing to speak. This can be stroking, cuddling, kissing, hugging, holding – or none of these, as some women do not want to be touched during labour.

Practising massage techniques regularly in the weeks before labour starts is important, as your partner should not be negotiating on the day about the speed (ideally slow and rhythmic) and intensity of how she wants the massage to be and what massage strokes she likes and does not like. You can read more on massage later in the book.

Words of encouragement

If you choose to use the hypnobirthing relaxation scripts and MP3 downloads included in this book you can use these in labour if wanted. Some women love hearing the scripts being read out by their partners, while others prefer listening to the MP3s. There is also an MP3 specifically for birth partners, to help you to prepare for your supporting role.

It is usual for a woman to have moments of self-doubt where she feels she cannot cope – calm words of encouragement may be helpful. Tell her how well she is doing, that she is birthing perfectly and beautifully and that it won't be long until you both meet your baby. Tell her how strong she is. But remember that keeping chat to a minimum is ideal, and keep quiet during a surge so she can focus on it.

Positions

Being gently active and encouraging your partner to get into upright, forward, open (UFO) positions can create almost a third more room for the baby to use.

If she is flat on her back this can hinder labour, as the sacrum at the lower back is not free to move and create more space. On her back she isn't utilising the powerful force of gravity to help her and she may feel less actively involved in the birth. Have a read of the positions for labour section and encourage your partner to try these out in advance.

Lower or raise the bed when you arrive in the room, as she will then be less tempted to lie down on it and can instead use it as a prop. If she is tired, then lying on the bed on her side is a good option. When on her side you can put pillows or a peanut ball between her legs to allow for a more 'open' position.

Encourage her to use a birth ball the right size for her (her knees should be a little lower than her hips, her feet comfortably steady on the floor). Birth balls usually come in 55, 65 and 75cm sizes. Kneeling, squatting and all-fours positions are also great for labouring in.

Breathing

Remind your partner to breathe slowly and deeply, with the out-breath as long as, or if possible longer than the in-breath for maximum oxygen supply to the mother, baby and the uterus.

Do some breathing practice together so you are familiar with how your partner looks when breathing in a relaxed manner. Calm breathing is also a great skill for you to have as a birth partner. If you notice she is starting to hold her breath or panic breathe, try co-breathing. Co-breathing is when you gently get her attention by holding her hands or shoulders or looking into her eyes and exaggeratedly breathe slowly and calmly in... and out... She can then mimic you and get back to her calm space and rhythm. If she doesn't want touch, you can count for her: 'Breathe in, 2, 3, 4 and out, 2, 3, 4, 5, 6.'

You can read more about breathing techniques, affirmations and visualisations later on in this book.

Think practically

Keep an eye on your partner and her surrounding area. Could she do with another pillow? Is she well supported and comfortable with relaxed shoulders, or is she tense and could do with a massage or a hug? Is she having regular sips of water? Pass her the water bottle to encourage this rather than asking her if she would like a drink.

Encourage her to empty her bladder every couple of hours as a full bladder can slow labour down.

Be her advocate. Take all questions in the first instance. This does not mean she cannot speak or engage with people, but when in active labour, particularly during a surge, she will need to stay focused. If you have something you are concerned about, quietly talk to the midwife about it out of her earshot, or at least wait until the surge has passed.

Control the environment

You can read about the importance of hormones and environment in this book. Get the room as dark as possible. Keep interruptions to a minimum. Organise the music if this is what she wants. What scents does she like? Lavender is soothing and calming; she may like to breathe in some lavender essential oil or lavender spray on a pillow or a cotton wool ball. If you're doing hypnobirthing, what scent have you been using during your practice? Use this.

Switch your phone off – you need to be focusing only on her. Perhaps you could set up a WhatsApp group on your phone in advance for family and friends and let them know you will update them via this as and when there is any news.

If you are getting yourself a drink or a cup of tea from the machine, offer your midwife one too. Chances are she has not had the time to have a break and would welcome a drink.

Handling questions and asking for information

Sometimes decisions need to be made in terms of your partner's labour/ progress, or in advance of labour starting. Unless it is a clear emergency, always take the time to ask for more information. Your partner will need to consent to any procedure or next steps, but you can help her get the information she needs to make that decision. Review the section on informed decision-making at the start of the book.

The questions below may be useful to ask if something is being suggested:

- 'Thank you for this information, please can you give us some time alone to discuss our options?'
- If time allows – so ideally before labour has started to give you time to read up – try 'I would be very grateful to read up on the evidence on XYZ – please can you point me to this to help us make our decision?'
- 'Is this an emergency or is my partner/wife/baby in danger? If not, we'd like to wait a bit longer to see how things progress and reassess in a little while.'
- 'How will what you are suggesting affect the labour/birth/our baby?'
- 'What other options are there?'
- 'Please can you explain that to me in a bit more detail?'

A useful acronym to help you think through what is being suggested is **BRAIN**: ask what are the:

- **Benefits** (of what is being offered)
- **Risks** (of what is being offered)
- **Alternatives** (to what is being offered)
- **Intuition** (what is your partner's intuition saying/what is her 'gut' feeling?)
- **Nothing** (is there time to do nothing for a moment/think it over a little or talk it through, perhaps with a consultant midwife or senior midwife?)

BRAIN is a useful tool for many situations, such as if your partner is being offered any intervention, like the suggestion of having her waters broken or induction of labour.

Being a birth partner can be hard work! Take care of yourself too by staying hydrated and eating.

Are you feeling concerned about being a continual support to your partner? Are you very anxious or worried about being a birth partner? Anxiety and stress mean you will be pumping adrenalin into her zone and at this time she should not be concerning herself with how you are doing. If you feel this way, consider having a second birth partner, someone who your partner feels safe and secure with and who will be a calming presence so you can duck out if things feel too much. If it's an option money-wise you could consider hiring a doula.

A birth partner's to-do list for labour

There are many things that you can do to help to encourage your partner into a relaxed state. If you are opting to do the hypnobirthing elements which feature later in this book you will find a breakdown there with suggestions on what to do and when. In early labour remember there is usually plenty of time. You can:

- Snuggle up and put on a funny DVD/comedy to watch – cuddles, laughter and relaxation produce oxytocin and endorphins and make us feel relaxed.
- Assuming surges are manageable, come up with other distractions for early labour – cook a meal together, play a board game, do crosswords, take a gentle local walk.
- Make sure your partner is gently active, but also resting and

conserving her energy.

- Make her a carb-heavy meal, but nothing too rich or creamy as this may make her feel sick.
- Play music, or listen to the hypnobirthing MP3s.
- Encourage her to stay hydrated with sips of water.
- Run a nice warm, candlelit bath.
- Have whichever essential oil/ blend she likes available for her to breathe in.
- Massage or hold her.
- When you arrive at the hospital be well versed in her birth preferences (birth 'plan') and make sure the midwife reads it.
- Be aware of your partner's health history so you can answer any questions if she wants you to do this.
- Ask to change midwife in the unlikely event you feel your birth preferences/plan is not being taken seriously or you do not feel supported. If this makes you feel awkward just remember that this day is just a shift in a midwife's career, but it is the only chance you will get to experience your baby's birth. Having someone with you who is not supportive of your wishes is not acceptable.
- When you arrive in your room, make it as dark as possible. Turn lights off and put blackout blinds up if you have them (you can get portable/ travel blinds to stick on windows).
- Remind your partner to empty her bladder every few hours as a full bladder can slow things down.
- Offer gentle, encouraging words, letting her know how amazingly well she is doing. Hearing your calm, familiar voice will help her feel supported.

A birth partner's to-do list for the third stage (delivery of the placenta)

- Keep your partner warm and relaxed. She may be shaky with adrenalin after the birth, which can delay the delivery of the placenta. Wrap a blanket around her.
- Encourage an all-fours or upright position.
- Suggest she empties her bladder if the placenta is slow in coming.
- Keep the lights low to maximise the hormone oxytocin, which is still needed.

- Make sure she has skin-to-skin with the baby, undisturbed, for at least an hour. If planning on breastfeeding, she can do this as it will produce a big hit of oxytocin, again helping to complete this last part of labour smoothly.

End-of-session summary

You've now read all about hormones and environment, place of birth and the birth partner's role. Below are some links for you to delve a bit deeper on these topics.

Hormones and environment

Some of these links are quite old, but don't let that put you off – the principle of undisturbed birth never ages.

- Lothian, Judith A. 'Do Not Disturb: The importance of privacy in labour' *Journal of Perinatal Education*, 2014. www.ncbi.nlm.nih.gov. Buckley, Sarah 'Undisturbed Birth', *AIMS Journal*, Vol 23, No.4, 2011. www.aims.org.uk/Journal/Vol23No4/undisturbedBirth.htm
- Barbeau, Beth 'Safer Birth in a Barn', *Midwifery Today*, 2007. www. midwiferytoday.com – this is an American article but makes for an interesting read.

Place of birth

If you have a few hospitals near you, do a bit of research on each one. They will all have a maternity section on their website and there may be an online tour video clip available. If at all possible, do a tour of each one so you get a feel for them all. Remember you can self-refer online if you want to change hospitals.

- Birthplace in England Research Programme, NPEU. Available at www. npeu.ox.ac.uk/birthplace
- www.nct.org.uk/sites/default/files/related_documents/Newburn%20 Birthplace%20in%20England%20p8-9%20Mar12.pdf

Birth partner's role

- www.nct.org.uk/labour-birth/dads-and-partners/choosing-your-birth-partners
- It would be great if you could do some massage and positions practice a few times a week and if possible, attend a good, relaxing pregnancy yoga course which focuses on breathing and positions for birth.
- 'Yoga in pregnancy enhances women's self-efficacy for labour and birth through repeated practice of a variety of pain management strategies and the telling of positive stories, magnified by the effects of yoga to lower somatic response further. The increased confidence and competence enables women to remain calmer, mobilise their pain management skills and take greater control of their labour.' Virginia Campbell, 'What is the impact of yoga for pregnancy classes on women's self efficacy for labour and birth?' www.maternityandmidwifery.co.uk/events/wp-downloads/midlands-2018/presentations/MMF_Midlands_2018_Presentation_Seminar_13_Virginia_Campbell.pdf

"

Let's talk about additional support (and what to pack!)

"

In the third session we talk about:

- The benefits of hiring a doula and what a doula does and doesn't do.

- Independent midwives - what are the benefits of hiring one, can you have an independent midwife alongside NHS appointments, and what packages of care can they offer?

- We'll also take a look at what to pack in your hospital bag and when to get this done by.

Chapter seven

Doulas – what are the benefits?

→ A doula is usually a non-medically trained birth professional, though of course there are some midwives who leave the profession and become doulas. A doula will be knowledgeable about the hospital you are giving birth in and will be familiar with their policies. She will provide continuous, non-judgemental support for you and your birth partner. She is someone you will have met and spent some time with in advance so you know that you 'click', that you are on the same page and that you feel comfortable with her and confident in her ability to support you. Quite often women meet with a few different doulas before making their decision.

A doula's role is to be there for you and to help your birth partner if needed, but she won't take over your birth partner's important role and will instead be led by you both. She can advocate for you if you wish her to, but won't attempt to sway your decisions in any way. Unlike midwives who will need to change over shifts, a doula will not leave your side throughout your labour. She can be as actively involved as you wish her to be, for example helping with massage, positions and breathing, or she can keep out of the way until you feel you need her support.

What are the benefits of hiring a doula?

- She will be a constant presence – there is a lot of evidence that when a woman has a constant, familiar presence during birth, labour progresses better and she has less intervention.
- She will support you whatever your choices and wherever you choose to have your baby.
- Women who have continuous support are more likely to have spontaneous vaginal deliveries and report being more satisfied with their birth experience.
- Women who hire a doula are less likely to request pain relief and are less likely to have a caesarean birth.
- Labour may be a bit shorter.
- She can, along with your partner, communicate to your care providers during labour, allowing you to keep your focus within.
- She can explain what is going on to you or your partner if you are unsure about things.
- She can provide physical support along with your partner, such as massage, or helping you with movement and positions.
- If your birth partner is very anxious, she can take the pressure off him or her, reducing the adrenalin in the room and leaving you free to concentrate without worrying about your partner's needs or fears.
- If you choose, you can hire her postnatally too, for example to help with breastfeeding, taking the baby while you have a shower and possibly carrying out light household duties or preparing meals.

What won't a doula do?

- She will not undertake any medical tasks such as examinations or helping you to birth your baby.
- She will not give you medical advice or attempt to sway your decision-making.
- She won't change shifts during your birth, as a midwife may need to.

Of course, hiring a doula costs money, and depending on where you are in the UK or the world prices can vary significantly. In the UK some doulas-

in-training offer packages which are less expensive while they train –
these are called 'mentored doulas'. Some women may be able to access
support with funding. You can find out if you could be eligible by visiting
the website **doula.org.uk** or calling them for more information.

Chapter eight

Independent midwives

→ Independent midwives are fully qualified, self-employed midwives. They carry out the same checks and assessments as their NHS colleagues, but rather than caring for many women, they care for the same woman throughout her pregnancy, birth and postnatal period, being on call 24/7. They can also provide just postnatal care, or both antenatal and postnatal care. Appointments will be flexible and longer so a woman and her partner have plenty of time to talk through any questions they have. They are also available by phone for any problems or questions.

Research demonstrates many benefits of one-to-one care (called 'caseloading' or continuity of care in the NHS) but this care is not available in all areas of the UK. The benefits of one-to-one care are:

- Women are more satisfied with their birth and postnatal experiences.
- You are more likely to have a spontaneous birth.
- Women are less likely to be induced.

- You are less likely to have an episiotomy or assisted birth.
- There's a reduced chance of having a caesarean birth.
- You are more likely to have a shorter labour.
- Women require fewer pain-relief drugs.
- Breastfeeding rates are improved.

Although there are no guarantees in life, including birth, choosing an independent midwife increases a woman's chances of having a straightforward birth because independent midwives provide the all-important continuity of care.

Most independent midwives attend home births, but they can also attend planned hospital births. If they have a honorary contract with that hospital they may be able to provide clinical care (if not, they will attend as an advocate and birth partner). They will be there for continuity and to protect your space. They can attend you in early labour at home and help you decide when to go in. If you need to transfer in from a home birth to hospital your midwife will go with you, but usually her NHS colleagues will take over your care and she will stay with you in the capacity of a birth partner or advocate.

Like all midwives, independent midwives are regulated by the Nursing and Midwifery Council. However, they have more freedom to provide individualised care as they are less restricted by NHS guidelines and protocols. Their aim is to offer evidence-based care and the woman is the decision-maker.

There is of course a charge for their services, but you will likely be able to pay in instalments. A large chunk of their fee will be to cover their insurance costs, which are very high.

If you choose to book an independent midwife, this does not mean you cannot access NHS care. If you wish you can combine the two and accept the blood tests, scans and any emergency care required that the NHS provides.

Chapter nine

Hospital bag – what to pack?

 When thinking about what to pack in your hospital bag, consider your five senses: sight, hearing, taste, touch and smell.

- **Sight.** We've already covered this so you know that a dark environment is key. Sunglasses, eye mask, black out blinds.
- **Hearing.** Labour wards and birth centres may not be quiet and you will likely hear other women in labour. Pack noise cancelling headphones and a decent set of earplugs. How about a mini speaker and device to play your music playlist and hypnobirthing MP3s?
- **Taste.** Pack your favourite treats! As well as a selection of sweet and savoury items and plenty of drinks.
- **Touch.** Massage oils, soft and comfortable clothing.
- **Smell.** To counteract the smell of a hospital bring in your favourite essential oil to use (more on this later).

Some people like to pack two bags, one for labour and one for after the birth. It is a good idea for your birth partner to have their own bag too with a change of clothes, toiletries and snacks (so they're not taking your stash!). If you are driving to the hospital or birth centre you could then leave the postnatal bag in the boot of the car, to save room.

A good tip is to lay out everything for your labour and birth bags on the bed and ask your partner to pack them. That way he or she will know exactly where and what everything is.

Pack enough clothes for one day and night for you all, with a couple of extra outfits and bibs for your baby. You can then pack another bag with 2-3 nights worth of items for you and the baby and leave this ready packed at home. That way, should you need to stay in longer than expected someone can pop by and collect the bag for you, rather than them rummaging around trying to work out what you might want.

You will probably only use a few of the things that you bring, but as it can be hard to know what those things will be, packing for most eventualities is normal.

Even if you are planning a home birth it can be useful to pack similar bags, in case you need to transfer in to hospital at any point. It also makes it easy for your birth partner or any helpers to find the things that you need in the hours after the birth even if you are at home the whole time.

Here are some suggestions to consider.

Birth bag

- Your maternity notes, if they are still the hand-held version.
- Several copies of your birth preferences sheet – you can stick one up on the wall too (bring sticky tack if you want to do this).
- A TENS machine with spare batteries and spare pads if you're planning on using one.
- Food – a selection of sweet and savoury items for you and your birth partner as it's hard to know what you might fancy. If you like bananas, these provide good energy, as do dried fruits. Food for after the birth is good too, just in case it's the middle of the night and nothing is open.
- Sports cap water bottles or bendy straws so you can easily stay hydrated whatever position you are in.
- Phone charger – if you use your phone as your camera this is especially important for those first pictures!

- Important phone numbers written down, in case the phone runs out and you are unable to charge it.
- Camera if you're not planning on using your phone.
- Toiletries.
- Ear plugs.
- A plain carrier oil or pregnancy massage oil for massages or putting a few drops of whatever scent you like (providing it is safe to inhale or have on your skin during labour) onto some fabric or a cotton wool ball to aid relaxation.
- A small portable speaker and a device to listen from (fully charged mobile phone or laptop) for your playlist and/or hypnobirthing MP3s.
- Eye mask, black out blinds.
- Water spray to keep cool.
- A small battery-operated/hand-held fan.
- A loose, comfortable change of clothes for you.
- Flannels soaked in water and frozen separately in sandwich bags. You can then take them out and once they've defrosted a little use them on the back of your neck to cool you down. Flannels can also be used as warm compresses by the midwife to help to protect the perineum.
- A hot water bottle – some women find warmth comforting.
- Dressing gown.
- Slippers.
- Socks.
- Flip-flops for the shower (non-slip!).
- A nightdress or big T-shirt.
- Lip balm – gas and air can make your lips feel dry.
- Hair band. If you have long hair, you might want it tied up.
- Your own pillow (or even just the pillow case, which could then be put on the hospital pillow). The familiar scent of home will be very comforting and far more comfortable than the starchy hospital ones. Use non-white cases so the staff know the pillows/cases are yours. You could also use a large T-shirt for this purpose.
- Wipes for a quick freshen-up.
- Toiletries for a longer freshen-up! Treat yourself to a luxurious soap or shower gel. Just brushing your teeth can help to refresh you.
- A big towel.

Postnatal bag

- Loose comfortable clothing for going home in.
- Nursing bra and breast pads.
- Maternity pads for postnatal bleeding (more on this later) – you will likely need around 3-4 packets of these as they will require changing around every 2-3 hours for the first couple of days or so.
- Large, comfortable cotton underwear.
- Hairbrush.
- Pyjamas/something comfortable to relax in.
- Clothes for your baby such as a hat, a couple of all-in-one stretchy outfits, a cardigan, a couple of vests. The current recommendation is no hat for the baby while the baby is indoors. Additionally, the secretions and smell of the top of the baby's head promote oxytocin production, which in turn helps you birth the placenta and promotes breastmilk production.
- A night shirt that opens at the front for easy skin-to-skin contact with your baby and for ease when feeding them.
- Baby blanket and/or snowsuit if the weather is cold. Remember to remove bulky clothing before putting your baby into their car seat. If it is cold, you can tuck a blanket over the car seat straps once they are secured correctly.
- Socks and/or booties (depending on the weather).
- Nappies.
- Car seat in the car, already practised with or installed and ready to go! It is well worth getting your car seat checked to ensure that it is fitted correctly, as many are not and are therefore useless. There are independent car seat specialists, or sometimes local councils offer a free car seat checking service.

It's great to get your bags packed and ready by 36 weeks, but I say the earlier the better as once it's done you can just forget about it!

End-of-session summary

We've now covered the role of a doula, independent midwives and what to pack in your hospital bag. As ever, I invite you to do your own research on these topics, and below are a few links you may find useful reading to get you started.

Doulas

- Evidence Based Birth. 'The Evidence for Doulas'. Available at evidencebasedbirth.com/the-evidence-for-doulas www.doula.org.uk/what-doulas-do
- *Why Doulas Matter* by Maddie McMahon, Pinter & Martin, 2015

Independent midwives

- www.imuk.org.uk
- www.nct.org.uk/pregnancy/choosing-independent-midwife
- www.rcm.org.uk/news-views-and-analysis/news/one-to-one-care-backed-by-study

Hospital bag

- www.nhs.uk/conditions/pregnancy-and-baby/pack-your-bag-for-birth
- www.nct.org.uk/labour-birth/deciding-where-give-birth/giving-birth-hospital/hospital-bag-checklist-what-do-i-need-take

"

Let's talk about physical skills for labour

"

In the fourth session we talk about:

- Physical skills to help you in labour, starting with positions for labour - what are the positions that will give your baby the most amount of room to be born and will help things to feel more manageable?

- Breathing - there are many different breathing techniques to try out for the first and second stage of labour, and we look at why learning this skill is so important.

- Last but by no means least, we discuss a variety of massage techniques to aid comfort, and which essential oils are safe to use.

Chapter ten

Positions for labour

→ Before we get into the benefits of being upright and active for labour and birth, I'd like to mention something called 'optimal foetal positioning' (OFP). This is when a woman uses her position and how she sits when pregnant to possibly help encourage the baby into a position where the back of their head is at the front, facing forward, rather than posterior or 'back-to-back' (meaning the baby's head and back is facing the mother's back).

A posterior baby isn't in a wrong or bad position. For example, perhaps the shape of your pelvis means that this is the position your baby chooses.

Quite often, if a baby's position is posterior, or back-to-back, this can mean the mother has several days of on-off labour, making her overall labour slower. She often experiences back discomfort in between surges, meaning she cannot rest in between them, which is tiring. The baby will then need to turn to be born, which can sometimes take a long time. They don't always manage to do this and may need a little help out via an assisted birth.

There is not currently any robust evidence that being mindful of our position when pregnant encourages a baby into a certain position. However, some healthcare professionals suggest the following ideas when going about your day as a way to attempt to encourage your baby into a head-down position, with their back to your front or left side before labour starts.

You may also find that some of these positions and ideas help with back discomfort in the latter stages of pregnancy, as well as during labour.

If this is something you'd like to look into you could try the following:

- Being more active, assuming it's safe for you to do this. For example, try getting off the bus one stop earlier, swimming, pregnancy yoga, walking.
- Avoiding positions where you slouch, like sitting on a super soft chair or sofa that encourages you to lean backwards. The back of the baby's head is the heaviest part of the body meaning gravity could encourage this part to go towards your back – the lowest point.
- Try sitting on a dining room chair which is faced backwards (you can add a pillow to lean on for comfort), or sit on a birth ball to watch TV. Some women bring birth balls into their workplace to sit on and find that this helps to relieve back pain. The position to adopt is one where your knees are slightly lower than your hips so that your pelvis is tipped forwards, feet flat and steady on the floor.
- Adopt an all-fours position for a few minutes a day. This is also a good position to relieve back discomfort when pregnant and during labour.

Positions for labour and birth

Many people when asked to visualise a woman giving birth will picture a woman flat on her back for both labour and birth. This is usually how birth is depicted on TV, in films and pretty much everywhere!

In hospitals the bed usually takes centre stage, and when the woman gets on it she goes from being active to being still – becoming a passive patient. Some midwives may prefer a woman to be on the bed, and sometimes women may think they are expected to be on it. However, it is always your choice where and how you labour and give birth and you should be free to move around and get into whatever position you want. This is where your birth partner can step in, if necessary.

Being flat on your back and immobile during labour can make your surges feel much more intense. You may also feel helpless, as if labour is happening to you rather than you being actively involved in it. When you lie flat on your back the vessel which carries blood into your heart is restricted due to the weight of the uterus restricting the blood flow. Reduced blood and oxygen supply can lead to your baby becoming distressed, requiring intervention. If you are tired, side-lying can be beneficial. You can also give birth on your side. Your partner may help you and the midwife by raising your outer leg.

You could consider asking your birth partner to raise the bed when you get into your room so you can lean over it and use it as a prop, rather than being tempted to lie back on it. Or you can kneel on the bed itself over a pile of cushions or a bean bag. You can also lower the bed, put some padding on the floor (gardening knee pads are good for this) and kneel down, leaning onto the bed with pillows.

The following images show how a woman's position can restrict or create space within the pelvis.

The sacrum is a triangular bone in the lower back, at the bottom of the spine. It is slightly mobile and during the birth process it actually moves a little to allow the head past. Being upright and off your back in labour can create up to one third more room in the pelvis.

In this squatting position you can see that the sacrum is free and able to move back to widen the pelvic space.

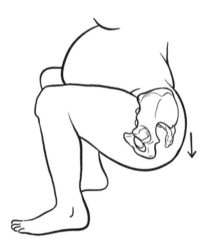

When a woman is in the semi-sitting position, her body weight rests on her coccyx and the pelvic space is reduced.

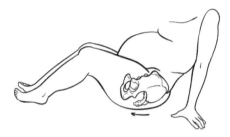

When a woman is in the reclining position the sacrum is immobile and the pelvic space narrows.

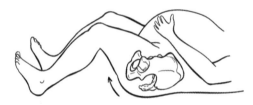

What are the benefits of upright positions in the first stage?

- More efficient surges.
- You feel more involved in your birth.
- The baby has a better oxygen supply.
- Movement is a good distraction for the mother.
- Birth partners can access your back or shoulders for massage.
- Squatting and all kneeling positions increase the diameter of the pelvic space.
- You make use of the powerful force of gravity.
- Swaying, rocking or circling on a birth ball, walking and going up and down the stairs sideways or two at a time (assuming there is no pelvic girdle pain present) may help your baby get into a good position for birth.
- Upright positions may shorten your labour and reduce the use of an epidural or having a caesarean birth.

What are the benefits of upright positions in the second stage?

- It may shorten the second stage.
- Fewer instrumental births (use of forceps and ventouse) and fewer episiotomies (surgical cuts to the perineum).
- Your birth partner can easily give you massage and hugs.
- The use of a ball in the second stage is thought to be supportive, providing counter-pressure on the perineum and helping the baby descend during second-stage pushing. It can also maximise pelvic capacity, though of course you'll need to be off the ball to actually give birth.
- Giving birth lying laterally (on your side) has been shown to have a protective effect on the perineum.

Some ideas for positions in labour/birth

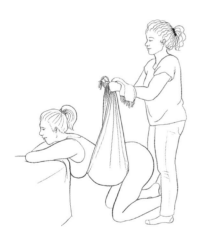

You can use a long scarf to fully encase the woman's bump and gently move the material from side to side to give a soothing, rhythmic motion of the pelvis, helping to relax the woman and providing movement. Look up 'Rebozo' for more information on this - and to see other positions in which Rebozo can be used.

If you're unable to get access to a pool to labour in you can stand, squat or kneel in the shower and have the water cascading down your back.

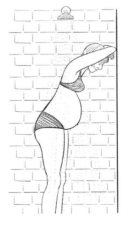

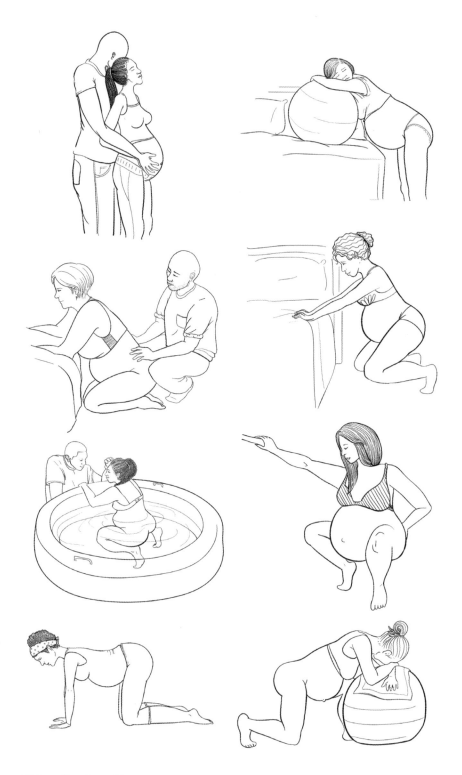

This collection of images shows some of the positions you may find useful or comfortable during labour.

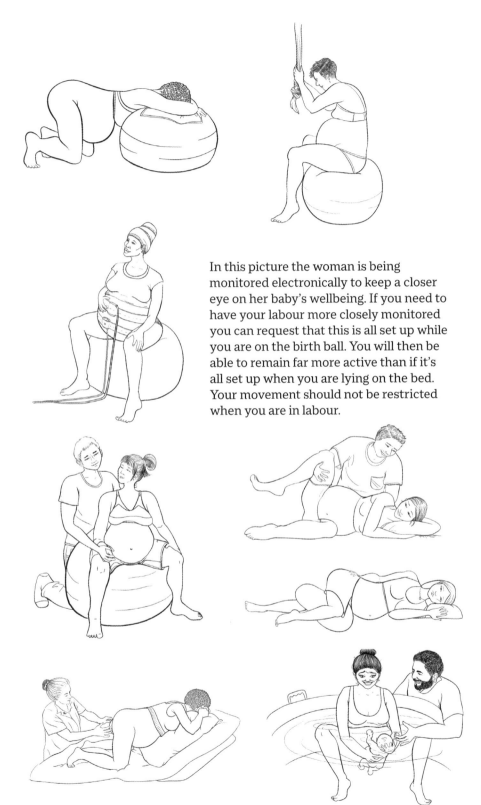

In this picture the woman is being monitored electronically to keep a closer eye on her baby's wellbeing. If you need to have your labour more closely monitored you can request that this is all set up while you are on the birth ball. You will then be able to remain far more active than if it's all set up when you are lying on the bed. Your movement should not be restricted when you are in labour.

85

Chapter eleven

Breathing in labour

→ The Autonomic Nervous System (ANS) controls our body's involuntary functions like keeping our heart beating, controlling blood pressure and keeping us breathing all without us having to think about it. It is divided into two parts – the sympathetic nervous system ('fight or flight') and the parasympathetic nervous system ('rest and digest') which gets things back to normal after any danger or stress has passed, calming and relaxing the body.

Slow, relaxed, rhythmic breathing activates the relaxation response of your parasympathetic nervous system – it's an inbuilt relaxation response. It causes your nervous system to change its state into one of calm, soothing both the body and the mind.

For the muscle fibres of your uterus to function well and efficiently they need a good blood and oxygen supply. Slow, calm breathing will help with this, keeping you focused and conserving energy.

Sometimes a woman in labour will tense her body and hold her breath during surges, which increases her adrenalin levels and reduces oxytocin.

This soon starts to makes her feel panicky and she greets the next surge with fear and anxiety, triggering the sympathetic nervous system. She continues to tense up and surges feel more uncomfortable. Due to the raised adrenalin the body assumes there is a threat to be managed so it starts the 'fight or flight' response. Blood is diverted from the uterus as this is not deemed a useful organ when faced with a threat. Even though the threat is imagined, the mind does not know this and it will think 'now is not a time to be giving birth!'. Blood will instead be directed to the arms, legs and brain to be useful for the 'freeze' 'fight' or 'flight' response.

Breathing becomes shallow, oxygen is decreased for you and your baby and it won't be long before you feel light-headed and out of control. This type of breathing cannot be sustained for long and quickly exhausts you.

Now that the uterus doesn't have oxygen and a good blood flow, it won't be long until it too gets tired, causing unnecessary pain in labour and making surges less efficient. Your hands and your jaw may clench tightly and shoulders tense up around your ears, making them feel tight.

If this sounds alarming, the good news is that there's a lot you can do to help to keep your breathing calm and in control, and your body relaxed, during the active stage of labour.

- When you feel you no longer want to chat through your surges, this is the time to start your birth breathing – though of course you can start earlier if you wish to.
- Surges are like waves. They start off mild, slowly building up until they reach a peak of intensity lasting around 20–30 seconds, and then peter out down the other side. There is then a gap where no sensation is felt until the next one begins (unless the baby is back-to-back, when the mother may feel back discomfort in between surges. All-fours positions and back massage will help with this).
- When you feel the surge starting, a sighing out-breath can shake off tension that has built up or crept into your body (see the 'pre-surge body scan' in the hypnobirthing chapter to help with this).

You might like to try this out now as we go through it:

- Quickly assess your posture – where are you tense? Make every muscle relaxed and loose, like a puppet whose strings have all been released. Open your hands/palms: this signals relaxation. Relax your jaw – you can rest the tip of your tongue behind your front teeth if this helps.

- Rest your hands lightly on your belly with your fingers just touching.
- Closing your eyes can help take your focus within. Some women like to wear eye masks to help with this.
- Breathe deeply in through your nose, focusing on filling your lungs to their capacity, gently expanding your ribcage, and then send the breath into the belly, letting that too gently expand so the fingers are slightly moved apart, creating space for your baby in the uterus.
- When you have filled your lungs and belly comfortably, slowly let the breath out through a soft, slightly open mouth, releasing the air with no effort, elongating the out-breath.

Breathing in this way means it takes longer for the out-breath to complete than the in-breath, and this is important in keeping you calm. Sighing releases tension, so try slowly sighing out the out-breath to keep relaxed. If you prefer to breathe in and out of your nose as you find this more natural this is of course fine – as always, do what works best for you.

- Repeat these long, slow, deep breaths in and out until you feel the surge peter out, and if you wish you can end the surge with a short sigh, releasing any last bit of tension.
- Most women then prefer to breathe normally in between surges, but if you prefer to continue with the birth breathing that's fine.
- Focus on the present moment, not what's ahead. Tell yourself 'Right now I am breathing slowly and calmly through this surge'.
- Some women find visualisations, mantras and affirmations helpful. For example 'Breathing in relaxation, breathing out softness/tension/stress'. Or on the in-breath 'I am', and on the out-breath 'strong' – and so on. Tell your brain what you want your body to do, clearly and simply.

Here are some breathing techniques and ideas to try out:

- Use visualisations, such as imagining seeing your out-breath slowly being released. Using colour can help with this, as can imagining seeing your out-breath like you do on a cold day. Any visualisations around opening and softening may be a good focus as this is what you want your body to do.
- Breathe in deeply and say 'relax, relax, relax' to yourself on the out-breath.
- Saying the word 'yes' is surprisingly freeing! 'No' is such a closed word,

whereas mentally (or out loud!) saying 'Yes, I am doing great' or 'Yes, I am one step closer' or simply saying 'yes' repeatedly, slowly and calmly, feels empowering.

- Try counted breathing: breathe in, 2, 3, 4, breathe out, 2..., 3..., 4..., 5..., 6.... Pregnant women have reduced lung capacity, so do not feel disheartened if you cannot get much of a long out-breath when practising before your baby arrives. You may find that after around 36 weeks, as the baby engages in your pelvis, you have better lung capacity. Many women find with practice they're able to elongate their out-breath more, but don't force things so you feel uncomfortable. The breathing should feel pleasant and calming as you practise.

- Breathing 'through the body' can be accompanied by placing a hand over an area affected by pain or tension. As you slowly breathe in and out, imagine a warm or cool sensation flowing through the hand into the muscles of the body, soothing and dissolving away any unpleasant sensations. This is also useful as a self-help strategy for coping with panic attacks. If you ever feel panicky during labour, or at any time, you can rest the palm of your hand on your chest and imagine a warm glow spreading from the hand into the chest and heart area, dissolving any tension, and allowing breathing to become more comfortable and natural.

- Place your hand on your heart and breathe in and out slowly for five seconds (you can go for a bit longer on the out-breath if you wish). This can be a good way to focus on calming down your heart rate if you feel panicky.

- Try saying: 'I am' on the in-breath and 'calm/relaxed/strong' on the out-breath. Or on the inhalation say 'Strength/courage flows in' and on the exhalation say 'fear flows out'. Or try saying 'Breathing in, I sink deeper and breathing out, I float freely'.

- Place your hands on your bump and breathe 'through' your bump. This can help you to focus on expanding the breath deep into your belly and reminds you that your breathing is also helping your baby.

- Picture a rectangle or look at a door frame. Breathe in, 2, 3, 4 while looking at/imagining the shorter length and out, 2, 3, 4, 5, 6, while looking at/imagining the longer length. Repeat until the surge has ended.

- Place one hand on your belly and imagine you can breathe into the palm of your hand as you inhale, then gently release the belly and the breath on the exhalation.

- Imagine you're standing on a sea of strength and energy and as you breathe in energy rises up through your body until it reaches the top of your head and as you breathe out, a warm shower of relaxation and calm cascades over your head and down your body, washing away any tension with it.

- Take one surge at a time: each one is bringing you one step closer to meeting your baby.

Breathing for the second stage (the pushing, or breathing down stage)

The second stage of labour is all about your baby's passage into the world as they move downwards with each surge. For the second stage you might imagine your baby being nudged downwards by your powerful out-breath.

When your cervix is fully dilated (and assuming you do not have an epidural in place), at some point most women feel an irresistible urge to push or bear down. This is often a very instinctive stage of labour, so follow your body's lead: it knows what it's doing.

As you will feel a natural, powerful urge to push during this stage, it is best to avoid 'coached pushing' as it really is not needed. Coached pushing involves sustained breath-holding and being directed when and how to push, and you have probably seen it in TV dramas. 'Take a deep breath in, hold it! Put your chin to your chest and push! Push! Push!'. This is not recommended, unless there is a clinical situation. There is no evidence of any benefit to this technique and women should be encouraged to bear down based on their own preferences and comfort.

Coached pushing is disempowering and is associated with raised blood pressure and a reduction in your baby's oxygen supply. It is also exhausting, unpleasant, and may leave you feeling lightheaded. There is nothing wrong with pushing as you get the urge to do so. Often this feels really 'right' if you're following your body's lead to push and are responding to what your body is telling you to do.

You may like to take a deep, strong breath in through your nose and let the breath out through your nose (or mouth if you prefer), firmly but not excessively forcefully, still keeping the jaw loose. Focusing downwards towards your pelvic floor will help you to encourage your baby downwards. This type of breathing keeps you energised and maintains a good flow of oxygen. It can help to visualise how a coffee plunger gets pushed down in a cafetière and think of the out-breath operating like this and see your baby in your mind's eye moving peacefully down with each out-breath. You can visualise your out-breath moving down the back of your throat (perhaps similar to the Ujjayi breath for anyone who does yoga), all the way down your body towards your pelvic floor as a powerful but gentle force helping to nudge your baby on their journey into the world. It is more effective to get two or three short pushes/nudges in with each surge, rather than one long breath-holding push. You can also try making deep, low sounds while focusing downwards/towards your bottom. Keep your mouth and jaw relaxed.

If you've had an epidural, your midwife will normally advise you to delay pushing for up to one or two hours from the time you are fully dilated, as this gives your baby a chance to descend further into your pelvis. As an epidural numbs a woman from the waist down, it can be hard to know when to push – work with your midwife to find out what breathing techniques may help at this time. You can also try breathing into the top of a closed fist which may help to direct the breath downwards.

Most women make some noises when pushing – this is kind of unstoppable and it's perfectly normal during this expulsive stage of labour. Making sounds is freeing and helpful and should not be restricted in any way.

Below are some of the advantages to learning breathing techniques for labour and birth:

- This type of breathing triggers the parasympathetic nervous system.
- Increased oxygen levels for you and your baby.
- Helps keeps you calm and clear-headed, no matter what else is going on around you.
- Gives you something to focus on right now.
- Lowers your heart rate.
- Stabilises blood pressure.
- Conserves your energy during labour.
- Relieves stress.
- Stops panic breathing and breath-holding.
- Helps you to feel in control.
- Can be coupled with counting, affirmations and visualisations to make it even more powerful and effective.
- Is a great distraction tool.

Breathing and positive affirmations scripts are available in the appendix and can be streamed or downloaded at: www.baby-bumps.net/bookmp3s.

Chapter twelve

Massage in labour

→ Receiving massage during labour can be comforting and brings you closer to your birth partner. It is a way of communicating without words and a way for your partner to let you know they are there for you. Massage also stimulates endorphin and oxytocin production. Some essential oils are safe to use, diluted in a carrier oil, and there's more on this later. However, some women prefer not to be touched during labour and that is fine too.

Massage can relax muscles, lower blood pressure, stimulate circulation, reduce pain and help you to mentally relax. Practise massage techniques during your pregnancy so that when you are in labour your partner knows what you like, what you don't like and how much pressure and speed to use. Make sure that he or she is well versed in slow, rhythmic massage. You do not want to be negotiating this kind of thing on the day.

Any kind of touch can be comforting. Kissing, cuddling, hugging, holding and stroking are all great.

Massage of the back, shoulders, neck, legs and hands can feel good.

Massage of the feet can feel good too, even if this is not usually your thing. For feet the pressure should be firm or it will feel annoyingly tickly.

Light strokes are when your partner uses the backs or tips of his or her fingers to gently stroke you. Some women like this, others do not. If it irritates you, you can ask your partner to use their flattened palms rather than fingertips to stroke more firmly.

When labour becomes more intense, some women like to have a counter-pressure back massage during a surge. Partners can use their knuckles, thumbs, the heels of their hands or tennis balls to massage the lower back area. When using firm pressure it is important to avoid the spine and instead focus on the fleshier parts, such as the tops and sides of the hips and buttocks, or circle around the sacrum. You can also do self-massage with tennis balls by leaning against a wall and placing the balls behind you, exactly where you want them, and then rocking from side to side.

If you prefer not to have your body touched, having your face or hair stroked may be preferable, or having your hands massaged.

Rebozo (a long scarf)

This can be used both in between and during surges. Using a scarf or Rebozo, your birth partner or doula 'jiggles' your body, helping to create room for your baby, relaxing muscles and helping to release adrenalin. It can be done with the woman on all fours and a scarf is either held across her buttocks, or totally encasing her bump, and a steady jiggle back and forth is given whilst the partner holds each end of the scarf.

The birth partner can also use their hands to carry out this jiggling movement with the woman standing up, feet hip-width apart, and the partner rubs their hands back and forth and up and down on her hips and thighs. The movement should be rhythmic and feel good to the mother.

A quick internet search looking up 'Rebozo' and 'shaking the apples' will bring up images and video clips to help you and your partner to visualise how these techniques are carried out.

Essential oils

Essential oils are powerful substances and caution should be exercised when using them. Do not use essential oils if you have a medical condition, you have an infection, an allergy, a skin condition, a multiple pregnancy, placenta praevia, are on any medication or if your baby has a condition or is being specially observed, until you have spoken with your doctor. Essential oils should not be used if you have any vaginal bleeding or if your labour begins prematurely. Always exercise caution and, if in doubt, use a plain carrier oil such as grapeseed oil or cold-pressed organic sunflower oil for massage until you have had the chance to speak to your doctor or midwife.

If you use essential oils during labour let your midwife know in case she has a health condition or she is pregnant.

Oils that are suitable for maternity use are:

- Bergamot
- Black pepper
- Roman chamomile
- Clary sage (NOT during pregnancy – only during labour, after speaking with your midwife)
- Cypress
- Lavender
- Lime
- Mandarin/tangerine
- Neroli
- Sweet orange
- Eucalyptus
- Frankincense
- Geranium
- Grapefruit
- Peppermint
- Rose (after 34 weeks)
- Spearmint
- Ylang ylang

You can add a single drop of oil to a cotton wool ball and breathe this in. Discard it after two hours and get a fresh one if still wanted. Be aware that if you are doing this plus, for example, having an essential oil footbath, then you are doubling up on the amount of essential oils getting into your body.

If you want to enjoy oils via a vaporiser at home this should not be used for more than 15 minutes at a time. You cannot use a vaporiser on the labour ward or in the birth centre.

Clary sage can be used to help boost surges that have petered out. As

Denise Tiran states in her fantastic book *Aromatherapy in Midwifery Practice*, it is very important to speak to your midwife before using clary sage to discuss why the surges have petered out. Could it be because you are anxious or fearful, dehydrated, need some food, or is it because of the position of the baby? It is also important to note that it is not advised to use clary sage to help with surges when labour has been induced. You can talk to your midwife about potentially using this essential oil an hour after any drugs have been administered.

If you want to use essential oil blends (where 2–3 different essential oils are blended together), check with a qualified aromatherapist that the ones you plan to use are safe for labour, or buy a pre-blended pregnancy massage oil.

If you're not keen on massage during labour essential oils can be used with a foot bath, a warm or cold compress, face spray or as a mini 'roll-on' for your pulse points. It is important that the oils you use are safe and are diluted appropriately, so ensure you check with an aromatherapist or purchase pregnancy-safe blended oils.

If you have had an epidural, avoid lavender, ylang ylang and clary sage as these can lower blood pressure, and an epidural also lowers blood pressure. If you are given any medication or have any interventions during labour check with the midwife before using essential oils.

In labour avoid using oils on the front of the upper body as the strong smell may interfere with the baby's natural ability to locate the breasts for feeding after the birth.

Avoid teas made with parsley, sage and fennel during pregnancy.

Here are some massage techniques to try:

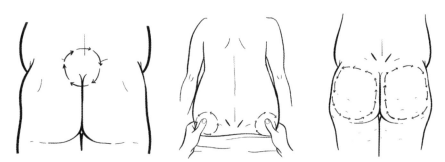

Massaging the sacrum firmly in a circular motion can feel great. You can use the heel of the hand, or even tennis balls – but these can give quite a strong pressure so go gently at first.

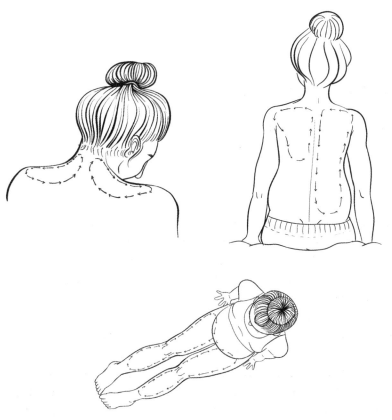

Sometimes it's not possible to get to the back, in which case a firm leg and/or foot massage can be good.

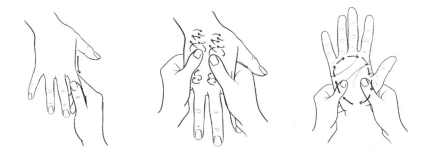

We can hold quite a bit of tension in our hands, and women often clench them during surges. Again, if the back cannot be accessed, a hand massage can be comforting. This is a suggested hand massage routine, but there are no real rules, so go with what you enjoy.

End-of-session summary

We've now looked at positions for labour, breathing and massage. Here's a recap and some suggestions for other preparation you can do.

Positions

Practise positions for labour using things around the house like your kitchen counter to lean on, your bed to lean over and so on. If you don't already have one, it's great to buy or borrow a birth ball and practise positions on it. Birth balls and gym balls are the same thing, just make sure it's an anti-burst one.

The more you practise the positions the more likely you are to use them on the day. They will also be invaluable when at home in early labour and for any back discomfort in the latter stages of your pregnancy.

Go onto YouTube and search for 'positions for labour' and include 'using a birth ball' and 'using a peanut ball' in a couple of the searches so you can watch how to use movement with and without a ball and then try this out at home.

Breathing

Practise breathing with your birth partner - this will enable them to help you, as well as helping them learn the techniques to keep calm on the day. Try out each of the breathing techniques within the breathing chapter – you may surprise yourself with which ones you like and use on the day.

Try this practice surge exercise with your birth partner or just by yourself.

In active labour, surges usually last around 50-60 seconds so for the purpose of this exercise, let's use 50 seconds.

1. Get a stopwatch or timer – most mobile phones have one in the clock/ alarm settings.
2. Sit with your birth partner and do nothing except count how many 'normal' breaths you do in a 50-second period. Breathing in then out is one breath. In and out again is two breaths, and so on.
3. Make a note of how many breaths you did in a 50-second period.
4. Reset the stopwatch.

5. Put on some relaxing music.
6. Start the stopwatch.
7. This time imagine you can feel a surge building so you greet it with a sigh and relax your whole body.
8. Get into one of the birthing positions, rock and sway.
9. Take a long, deep, slow breath in, and if possible, release a longer out-breath. Try counted breathing or a visualisation. You can include an affirmation too. Repeat this breathing until you have reached 50 seconds.
10. Have your partner massage you if they're around.
11. After 50 seconds is up note how many breaths you did.

Most people are surprised to note that second time around seems a lot faster! They usually report doing fewer breaths the second time, and find that it takes around 3-5 slow, deep breaths rather than the usual 10-15 normal breaths.

This exercise is a great way for you both to see the benefits of distraction in the form of visualisation, counting, affirmations, movement and music. It's reassuring to know that in around 3-5 breaths your surge will be finished and it will have been beautifully efficient, with great blood flow and oxygen for you and your baby.

Remember that the peak of the surge, when it is at its most intense, usually lasts around 20-30 seconds, which is pretty much 1-1.5 breaths in... and out.... You are now one step closer to meeting your baby.

Massage

Again, I invite you to go to YouTube and search for massage in labour. There are also lots of useful links on my padlet: padlet.com/jackiekietz/book

"

Let's talk about hypnobirthing

"

In the fifth session we talk about:

- Hypnobirthing. Here we'll take a look at the power of the mind and how you can harness this during pregnancy, labour and postnatally.

- We'll go through what hypnosis is, and isn't, and you'll learn how to use the powerful tool of self-hypnosis, which is a fantastic life-long skill. A wide range of hypnobirthing and mindset techniques will be covered in this session so you can try them all out in your own time and pick and choose which ones you feel fit you best.

- Included at the end of the book are 10 scripts, covering, among other things, caesarean birth, induction of labour and postnatal/general confidence. All the scripts are also available as MP3s.

- You can also read a selection of positive birth stories that cover a range of scenarios.

Chapter thirteen

Hypnobirthing

→ Giving birth is a huge physical feat, but your mind also has a big role to play. The power of the mind is a vast subject, but in this chapter we will look at the power of the mind for labour and birth.

When you find out you are pregnant, you may start taking vitamins, pay attention to your diet and stop drinking alcohol, to keep your body and baby healthy. But how many women think about giving their mindset a makeover?

Birth is a normal event. It is certainly hugely challenging – but it is generally very safe thanks to advances in hygiene and antenatal and postnatal care. However, I will take a bet that sadly most women are absolutely terrified of giving birth – and it is no wonder, when you consider what we have been fed about childbirth all our lives by media, friends and family.

How often do we see a positive birth on a TV show or in a film? Have you heard many positive birth stories from friends, or read many positive birth articles in magazines or newspapers? Why don't we ever read or hear about all the many straightforward, positive births which happen every day? Of course this is because they aren't newsworthy and as births like this are everyday occurrences they don't sell papers.

When you consider how birth is portrayed on TV and in the media, you probably think of something like this: a woman's waters break dramatically. She clutches her stomach in immediate agony. She is rushed to hospital, in great pain. She lies flat on her back in hospital, screaming and writhing around, while she is shouted at to 'Push! Push! Push!'. She is surrounded by people. The baby is 'delivered' by staff telling her what to do and usually her partner is shown as being a 'spare part'.

The problem is that unless you have given birth positively before or are lucky enough to have been surrounded by positive birth stories and images, these negative stories and images are the ones your mind will 'go to' when you are in labour, and this can dramatically affect how your body works. These negative images and birth stories plant seeds in your mind, creating a certain belief around how birth is. They chip away at your confidence in your ability to birth your baby, taking away trust and faith in your perfectly designed, incredible body.

Our beliefs and habits are very powerful and they dictate how we will respond to things – we respond in the way in which we are 'programmed'.

If a woman is very anxious about birth, thanks to the beliefs she has built up and stories she has heard since she was young, when she goes into labour she will experience automatic feelings of fear, that birth isn't safe, and so on, which will raise her adrenalin levels, setting off a chain reaction that can hinder and slow down labour as well as making things feel much more intense.

The good news is that there is a lot you can do right away to reboot and 'reprogramme' your mind. You can:

- Stop watching programmes that depict birth negatively. They fill your mind and thoughts with negative birth fodder that it will access and go to when it is your turn to give birth, increasing fear and anxiety.
- Watch positive births and hypnobirthing birth videos on YouTube – there are tons out there.
- Read up on and practise the techniques and exercises you'll find later in this chapter.
- Read positive birth stories on websites such as 'Tell me a good birth story'. You will find some positive hypnobirthing birth stories later in this chapter.

- Follow hypnobirthing accounts on Facebook and Instagram. The Instagram account linked to this book is baby_bumps_ hypnobirthing and the Facebook page is www.facebook.com/ HypnobirthingSouthLondon.
- Find out about your local Positive Birth meet-up group www. positivebirthmovement.org and borrow or buy birth preparation books that depict birth in a positive way.
- Close your ears to negative birth stories – don't be afraid to stop someone in their tracks if they are about to launch into telling you their birth story, by saying 'I'd love to hear your birth story once I've had my baby'. Of course, if you think their story will be super-positive, by all means listen.
- Choose some affirmations that you like from this book, from Pinterest, or just make up your own. Stick at least one up where you will notice it each day. Say it out loud, and say it in your head.
- Use visualisation to enhance your motivation, confidence and self-efficacy (your personal judgement about how well you can deal with a situation). All the top sports competitors use this powerful technique and there is more on visualisation later.
- Practise your breathing techniques every day, at random moments such as on a busy train or bus, or when you are feeling wound up by a colleague – as well as with your partner and before you go to sleep or get out of bed in the morning.
- Remind yourself (and have your birth partner remind you during labour) that you don't have to be on your back to give birth. Try out the positions included in this book. Practise them alone, with breathing, with your partner. If you practice them in advance you are more likely to use them on the day.
- If possible, as early as you can, attend a pregnancy yoga class or find a good free online one on YouTube. During these sessions you'll spend time practising birth positions, breathing and enjoying guided relaxations.
- Expand your knowledge – knowledge is power! After all, if you don't know your options, you don't have any.
- Understand how your amazing body works. Learn what helps and hinders labour. We cover all this in this book, but don't let that stop you from reading more and more.
- Mind your language. Tune into how you speak to yourself. Are you talking positively to yourself about your baby's birth?

What is hypnobirthing and hypnosis?

Some people may be put off by the word 'hypnobirthing'. If you know nothing about it the word may conjure up images of stage hypnosis where people are hypnotised to eat onions as if they were apples and to generally make fools of themselves. Stage hypnosis is done for entertainment purposes and is nothing like clinical hypnotherapy, self-hypnosis or hypnobirthing. In this book I take a cognitive behavioural hypnotherapy and mindfulness approach since this reflects my training as a hypnotherapist with the UK College of Hypnosis and Hypnotherapy.

Since hypnosis is a big part of hypnobirthing, let's start by exploring that a bit. Incidentally, all hypnosis is self-hypnosis as you are always in charge. When you listen to the scripts or MP3s this is simply guided self-hypnosis.

There's nothing magical about hypnosis. It's a collaborative process where you actually do most of the 'work' by relaxing, thinking positively and going along with what is being suggested. Hypnosis is an ordinary process, not an altered state of consciousness – and you are responsible for the responses you get.

It is something you've probably experienced many times already, but you've not called it hypnosis or self-hypnosis. For example, you may have been deeply absorbed in a film or book to the extent that it brings about a physical and emotional reaction of some kind.

We are always giving ourselves suggestions, sadly often negative ones which limit us. If you suffer from worry or rumination – focused attention on things that worry you – the good news is that you are already an excellent hypnotic subject! You already know how to lose track of time, become less aware of your surroundings and elaborate on the content of your negative thoughts in great detail, often for many hours. It could be said that you are already an expert in self-hypnosis since you have written your own 'negative' hypnotic scripts and have become imaginatively involved with them.

The good news (again!) is that you can rewrite the story of your thoughts and make them into something positive – more on thoughts later.

During hypnosis we focus only on positive suggestions. Truly wanting a suggestion to be effective and expecting it to be so is a powerful combination, like nurturing the seeds of our mind. If you do not engage in the process – with your imagination, absorption, thoughts and feelings –

no hypnosis occurs.

When you use self-hypnosis (which we'll cover later), listen to the scripts or MP3s featured in this book, or visit a hypnotherapist, you're allowing yourself to be guided by the suggestions within them (or by the hypnotherapist's words) by using your imagination to bring about positive thoughts, feelings and emotions around labour and birth. You are mentally rehearsing how you wish to react and behave during labour. You're simply opening your mind, allowing it to become suggestible, by relaxing and being attentive to the ideas being suggested. If you're able to become engrossed in a film, some music or a TV show, then there is no reason why hypnosis cannot work for you. It's just a simple but powerful way of rehearsing future behaviours in a positive manner.

Time seems to pass in an illogical way during hypnosis, just like when you get engrossed in something and suddenly you look up and realise it's late – this is due to the mental/imaginational absorption which takes place during hypnosis.

Hypnosis is safe and no one has ever got 'stuck' in hypnosis. There is no controlling of the mind, in fact quite the opposite: no one can make you accept the suggested ideas, nor can they force you to use your imagination to respond to the suggested events. You are always in control and you get back what you put in. The more you can 'get into' the suggestions, the more real it all becomes for your mind and the more likely you are to 'act it out', as per your previous rehearsals, on the day.

Hypnosis is not:

- The same as relaxation – though the two go wonderfully together and relaxation is a great 'side effect' of hypnosis.
- A sleep-like trance – hypnosis does not have to be accompanied by relaxation, it can be accompanied by alertness and energy. The word 'sleep' is sometimes used as part of the induction (an induction is a set of instructions given before the main body of the relaxation/hypnosis begins) – this is because of tradition, and because it can help to bring about the body's relaxation response. A person may feel so relaxed during hypnosis that they feel sleepy, but that's different to actually being asleep.
- Dangerous – but it is important to ensure you don't have any contraindications to hypnosis before embarking on it (please see below).
- Giving up your power – hypnosis can be stopped at any time simply by opening your eyes.

Contraindications to hypnosis

Hypnosis/self-hypnosis is just as safe as doing meditation or relaxations and is generally very good for your mental and physical health. However, please do not participate if you have a history or diagnosis of psychosis, psychiatric issues, clinical depression, epilepsy or you know of any other medical reason that might affect you. A simple rule of thumb would be to check with your GP/doctor first if you have any medical or mental health conditions, or have had in the past, before using hypnosis/self-hypnosis. Do not undertake hypnosis when under the influence of alcohol or drugs.

Only embark on any hypnosis practice when you are in a place where it is safe for you to relax and you do not need to be alert and aware of your immediate surroundings. After emerging from hypnosis give yourself some time to come back to the present and re-orientate yourself before driving a car or operating any machinery.

What is hypnobirthing?

Hypnobirthing is effective, logical antenatal preparation for birth that involves:

- Hypnosis/self-hypnosis via MP3s or having your partner read out scripts.
- Learning how to use self-hypnosis as a standalone technique so you can use this fantastic skill for life, without needing to rely on having access to MP3s.
- Easy to learn techniques to work with your breath.
- Understanding how you can use hugely beneficial hypnotic cues/triggers and post-hypnotic suggestions.
- Guided relaxations.
- An understanding of the power of the mind and the mind-body connection.
- Developing an understanding about the powerful effect of language on the mind and body during labour.
- Positive affirmations.
- Using visualisation.
- Learning how to release fears.

All this comes along with antenatal education, which we've already covered, on:

- The physiology of birth.
- Physical skills such as breathing, massage and movement.
- Understanding what helps and hinders labour and what you can do to help yourself.
- The birth partner's important role.
- Informed decision-making and an understanding of your options and choices during labour and birth.

So hypnobirthing is a complete antenatal education and preparation in and of itself, combined with some very practical, useful and powerful elements. You can think of it as birth education along with a mindset-reset or overhaul of how you view and respond to birth.

Women who practice hypnobirthing frequently report that they are able to relax and enjoy their pregnancy and feel more positive preparing for labour and birth. They enjoy listening to the guided relaxations and learning to trust their bodies. Women already 'know' how to give birth – it is in our DNA – but sadly, it is common for faith and trust in the process to have been lost along the way. Hypnobirthing gives women and their birth partners a set of tools and techniques that can help them to use their already present, natural birthing instincts.

The specific practice of breathing techniques and changed mindset can often result in a more comfortable birthing experience, with couples reporting that they felt calmer and in control, however their birth unfolded and including when it didn't go to 'plan'. Hypnobirthing has become very popular, with many women using the techniques. Some midwives now train in the method too, which is fantastic.

Hypnobirthing is not necessarily about removing pain, but rather it is about reframing it and understanding how your body is working hard to birth your baby. The breathing and mindset practices help to allow you to let go and give yourself over to your body, rather than fighting against it or resisting the power of your surges.

While some women report that they only experienced tightenings or pressure during their labour, other women report that they did feel pain, but that they did not feel out of control or frightened by it. They understood what its purpose was, that their body was working hard to bring their baby to them rather than something wrong or bad happening.

Where possible, it is best to start your hypnobirthing preparation early in your pregnancy, with most women starting around 20–32 weeks of pregnancy. This is to enable lots of repetition in order to embed a different mindset around birth. However, if you come to hypnobirthing later than 32+ weeks, it is important not to be put off – you will just need to commit yourself and intensify your practice, rather than building it up slowly.

Advantages of hypnobirthing

Hypnobirthing techniques help you to relax, which, along with the techniques practiced in advance and used on the day, will mean:

- You are going to be breathing deeply and calmly, which increases oxygen to you and your baby.
- You will be activating the parasympathetic response of 'calm and connection' as opposed to 'fight or flight', ensuring the uterus, placenta and baby will have a good blood supply.
- Surges are likely to be more efficient.
- Endorphin production, the body's natural and super powerful painkiller, will be enhanced.
- You and your partner will feel empowered.
- Your experience of childbirth will be improved.
- Your birth partner will be very much involved and have an important role.
- You may find you do not require any pain medication.
- You are informed and understand how your body works in labour.
- Women report feeling calm and in control, whatever turn their birth takes.
- There are no harmful side effects to you or your baby – in fact babies benefit from the increased oxygen thanks to the regular, deep breathing.
- Practising hypnobirthing during pregnancy will often mean that you are able to feel more positive approaching the labour and birth. You will have a tool kit to enable you to deal with challenges or 'wobbly' moments, which means that you are able to enjoy your pregnancy without unnecessary fears hanging over you. All of these relaxed feelings will also benefit your baby greatly.

- When you practise relaxation (all the book's MP3s include this) once a day you will usually find you feel more relaxed in general.
- Parents report that they enjoy a little time out a few times a week to focus on the pregnancy, baby and each other.
- You can also practise alone if you prefer this or if you do not have a specific birth partner.
- You will learn the valuable life skill of how to do self-hypnosis.

It can be tempting to over-schedule and pack things in, particularly in the last trimester, which is often the most tiring part. Your hypnobirthing practice will give you time to focus on yourself and your inner preparation. Your hypnobirthing practice is a way of scheduling in time to relax and it's a lovely way to connect with your baby and your partner during such a busy time in your lives.

Potential disadvantages of hypnobirthing

- Consistent time and effort is required in order to get the full benefits of hypnobirthing – but this is often described as relaxing, enjoyable and positive, so is this really a disadvantage?
- If you choose to do a course this costs money, but many women successfully practice hypnobirthing by reading books and listening to scripts or MP3s.
- You may not have a practitioner in your area, but a live online course using a platform such as Zoom works well (see **www.baby-bumps.net** for this option).
- Sometimes women feel hypnobirthing didn't work for them, or that it only helped them for part of their labour and they feel disappointed about this.

As well as using hypnosis/self-hypnosis, I like to include other techniques and I describe these below, starting with self-hypnosis.

Self-hypnosis

While MP3s are fantastic tools for you to use now and during labour, it's a great skill to learn how to do self-hypnosis. Once you've learned this valuable technique, you are no longer reliant on having to have headphones and MP3s at the ready. This is wonderfully empowering and you can use it to help you throughout life – in times of stress, when you need a confidence boost, when you're feeling overwhelmed in early parenthood, or for healing or recovery purposes.

Below is a sample self-hypnosis technique. I recommend listening to the general relaxation and confidence/postnatal MP3 before trying this out so you first get a feel of classic hypnosis.*

- To prepare, first of all choose a trigger word that will help you to relax such as 'relax' or 'calm' and repeat it in your mind at the end of each deep breath.
- Then pick an affirmation or positive suggestion that you can silently repeat to yourself, such as 'Each day I grow more calm, confident and strong'.
- Next think of a relaxing scene such as lying on a beach or sitting in a beautiful garden.
- Finally, think of the body as being divided into three sections which you will relax in turn. 1) from the waist down to the feet 2) the chest, back and arms and 3) the head and neck.

Now you have prepared, try the self-hypnosis routine (it takes about 10–15 minutes). Read it through a few times to memorise it:

1. Begin by taking a good, deep breath and allowing the eyes to close. Take a moment to unwind and focus on your breathing. Clear your mind and make yourself comfortable.
2. Take a deep breath in and hold it for about 10 seconds. Letting out a sigh, repeat your trigger word to yourself as you relax your whole body. Allow your breathing to return to normal for a few moments as you relax the body.
3. Breathe in again, in the same way. Relax the lower body more deeply, from the waist down to the feet, as you exhale and repeat the trigger word.
4. Another deep breath, relaxing the chest, back and arms deeply as you exhale.
5. And once again, deeply relaxing the head, neck and face as you breathe out.
6. Finally, to catch any remaining tension, deepen the relaxation of

* Technique courtesy UK College of Hypnosis and Hypnotherapy. **www.ukhypnosis.com**

the whole body again as you breathe out. If you want, you can also imagine using this breath to expel any mental or emotional tension.

7. Smile to yourself gently – notice pleasant relaxation can increase when you smile to yourself.

8. Take a few moments to settle and allow your breathing to return to normal and the mind to become empty, tranquil and quiet. Scan the body, looking for any areas where tension remains or has returned. Imagine it as a puff of coloured smoke being blown away by a soothing breeze. Smile to yourself again.

9. Now imagine yourself at the top of a flight of stairs or steps. At the bottom is your relaxing place (the garden, beach or whatever you came up with). Slowly descend the steps one at a time counting from 10 down to zero as you do so. Imagine yourself sinking down deeper into a wonderful state of hypnosis with each step you take.

10. When you arrive at the bottom of the steps picture yourself entering your relaxing scene. Take a few moments to try to get a feel for the scene, take note of the colours you can see and the sounds you can hear. Allow yourself to let go completely and enjoy the pleasant feelings of physical relaxation and mental calm. Again, gently smile to yourself.

11. Now repeat your affirmation to yourself slowly, until you feel it taking hold. Remember to be aware of your imaginary tone of voice, mean what you say, get it sounding just right. When finished, take your time to settle again and to enjoy the feelings of calmness, relaxation and confidence which your affirmation has given you.

Optional – situation rehearsal: Imagine being in your target situation. Imagine it as if it is happening right now, really imagine being in the scene – take all the relaxation and calmness into that scene by repeating your affirmation to yourself in that scene. Go through it for 30 seconds. Imagine that your positive belief is growing stronger and stronger as you go through the scene. Imagine handling the scene in a more effective way. Let the scene go. Then repeat step 11 (or steps 10–11). Repeat this sequence five times. Finish with repeating your affirmation five times, smiling to yourself and really getting into the meaning.

● When you're ready, count from one up to five to emerge. Open your eyes, and give your arms and legs a shake.

How do you feel?

Awareness of thoughts: stopping, switching, changing them

Our thoughts are very powerful and they have an impact on our bodies and emotions. Stopping negative thoughts in their tracks can help limit and prevent unwanted internal negative self-talk and chatter. Sometimes we can be our own worst enemy with the way we talk to ourselves. Our thoughts don't matter, but how we respond to them does.

Write down the thought... develop an alternative more helpful thought... practice repeating it... Then spot it, stop it (from going onto the next thought but not suppressing the original thought), relax and switch onto your helpful thought.

An example:

- "I'm not going to cope with labour.... it's going to be horrible... STOP"
- Relax
- Repeat "I can handle this, my body knows what to do, I can cope... I breath and relax and accept..."

Writing out thoughts forces you to think about and critique the thought or problem, aiding clear thinking as well as helping you to become aware of your thoughts. So whenever you have a negative thought about your birth, write it down exactly as it is. That way you get to view it and it becomes exposed and weakened. It has also now moved out of your head so it is no longer rattling around in there, taking up space and energy.

You can then jot down how that thought is detrimentally affecting you – applying rationale and showing yourself there's little value in continuing such negative thoughts.

Finally, write down a replacement thought – something beneficial you could say to yourself instead. What would be a more helpful thing to tell yourself, or what would be the opposite of that thinking? This can then become an affirmation you use if you wish.

This little exercise will help you to spot/become aware of, dispute and restructure your thoughts. It is very powerful as it allows positive thoughts to dominate your internal dialogue and will hopefully start to reduce your negative internal chatter.

Here are some other ways you can help to manage your thoughts:

- Remember the difference between 'I believe' and 'I know' and consider your thoughts as hypotheses instead of facts
- Use a counter to keep a tally of negative thoughts – this will show you just how many habitual, repetitive negative thoughts you have each day and will help you to remember to stop them in their tracks.
- Change perspectives – if you're having a negative thought about being able to cope in labour imagine being in the shoes of someone who had a positive birth experience who therefore views things differently. What would they say to you? If you don't know anyone read some positive birth stories and imagine what that person would say to you.
- Picture your thoughts as puffs of cloud moving across the sky on a windy day - something transient, that only lasts for a short time. No need to respond to them – but also don't ignore them as this just prolongs them (try not thinking about a pink elephant and you'll see that this is exactly what you end up paying attention to!), just observe them.
- View your thoughts as background noise, white noise or like a radio playing quietly in a room.

We can't stop thoughts, but we can control what happens next by choosing not to worry, knowing the thought is just that – a thought, a scenario in the mind. Whether it is true or not, it will always be a thought.

Throughout the day practise observing your thoughts and thinking patterns in order to identify negative ones. Encourage yourself and be supportive in your thoughts about your ability to give birth. Talk to yourself kindly, as you would to a child or a good friend.

Releasing fear

We've covered how birth is depicted in our culture and within the media, meaning that women are understandably fearful of it. What we focus on tends to become our reality, so spending time before your birth releasing your fears and focusing instead on positive feelings and thoughts around birth is very beneficial.

You know from reading about some of the hormones in labour that fear can slow surges down and make things feel more uncomfortable than they need to be. And as we have seen, our thoughts have an impact on our bodies and emotions. For example, have you ever had a job you disliked, and found yourself getting that 'Sunday blues' feeling, when your heart literally sank at the thought of going to work on Monday? Or have you ever remembered an embarrassing situation and found yourself cringing and tensing up, as the feelings and physical sensations you felt at the time come flooding back to you? What about remembering a good night out with friends? Do you find yourself smiling or laughing to yourself when remembering the events of a fun evening?

These events aren't real right now – you're creating (or recreating) them in your mind, and your mind and body react by bringing up the relevant emotions and physical sensations regardless of whether it's a real event or not.

The idea behind processing and releasing fears around birth, and focusing on positive birth scenarios, is that this can help to create positive feelings, cognitions and a new neural pathway around birth. This new 'programming' means you are more likely to feel relaxed and have confidence and trust in your body on the day of your baby's birth.

The Fear-Pain-Tension cycle

In the 1930s, obstetrician Dr Grantly Dick-Read, author of *Childbirth Without Fear*, formulated what he called the Fear-Pain-Tension cycle – when we are fearful we become tense, and this tension causes pain. The pain then further fuels the fear, and so the cycle continues.

In preparation for labour and birth a woman's uterus has developed many more blood vessels than that of a non-pregnant woman, as the increased circulation is necessary for efficient muscular action. It needs plenty of oxygen and blood for it to work efficiently.

When we are tense and in pain we understandably feel panicky, and this panicky feeling can tip us into 'freeze, fight or flight' mode, which we have already covered, but below is a reminder of how this works.

Fight or flight is a very primitive response, designed to keep us safe from danger. When we are in the fight or flight state this enables us to be hypervigilant – looking for the threat, even if there is no real threat. Then:

- Our breathing becomes shallow and rapid, reducing oxygen, and our heart rate increases
- We feel nauseous
- We may feel sweaty and/or faint

- Blood drains away from the digestive system and non-essential organs for fight or flight (of which the uterus is one) and we may have a dry mouth

The result of all this is that birth is painful – and it is frightening because we are overly aware of our bodily sensations as a threat. This then becomes a vicious circle.

Dick-Read believed that when fear is removed, pain is reduced, or even removed altogether. There is no tension, which means that the uterus is able to work to its full capacity as it is perfectly designed to do.

While giving birth is no walk in the park, it does not need to be full of terror and tension. Spending time understanding how the body works in labour and what can hinder the process helps to prepare you, and spending time releasing any fear you have around childbirth will be very beneficial too.

Releasing fear is important for birth partners as well – if they can address their concerns about birth before the big day, they won't be bringing unwelcome anxiety, adrenalin and stress into the birth room.

What fears do you have around birth? Consider where they originate from. Are they actually your fears, or just things that you have heard along the way, or have been led to believe are true? Birth is generally very safe, but we tend to only remember and focus on the negative things we hear.

Spend a little time considering:

- Are you happy with where you are planning on giving birth or would you like to change this?
- Do you feel concerned or overwhelmed about any particular issues?
- Are you worried about lack of support during or after the birth? If so, who else can you call on? Is a doula an option?
- Is your partner on board with your birth wishes? Again, if not, is a doula or additional birth partner an option?
- Do you have past negative experiences to call upon?
- Do you recall a negative birth that you read about or saw on TV that has particularly stuck in your mind?
- Can you remember details from a friend's negative birth story which is sticking in your mind and making you worry?*
- Has a friend or family member had a difficult birth?*

Remember – these are not your stories!

It may feel easier and more comfortable to try to block out these concerns, but acknowledging them will help you to work through them and release them. Talk through them with your partner or a friend. You can also arrange to speak with a senior/consultant midwife if you have very specific or personal fears and they may be able to refer you on to a specialist team to help with this.

If any fears are linked with a past birth, ask to go through your notes with the consultant midwife to help you understand what happened – and why – in a safe and supportive space. You can discuss how best to try to ensure that things will be different this time and come up with a birth 'plan' that you feel happy with and are supported with. Try to release as much fear as you can before your birth.

Once you have identified any fears, where relevant, you can try the following:

- Write your concerns down, whether they are about birth or anything else that you want to release. Read them out, then tear them up into tiny pieces and throw them away.
- Visualise putting all fears into the basket of a hot air balloon. See yourself setting it free. Watch it float away until it is a tiny dot, then gone – taking the now-vanished fears with it.
- As each fear comes up, see it as a cloud leaving your head, floating upwards, drifting away, until you can see it no more.

You may also like to try this short, visual relaxation, which appears in *The Science of Self-Hypnosis: The Evidence Based Way to Hypnotise Yourself* by Adam Eason:

- Get comfortable, somewhere where you won't be disturbed for a short while. Slow down your breathing and say the word 'soften' or 'relax' (or another word of your choosing) to yourself as you imagine and feel the muscles of your body doing just that.
- Imagine going deeper into this softness and relaxation by imagining walking down some stairs. Or you could try counting downwards and backwards from 100–0, telling yourself that each number takes you deeper into this wonderful relaxation.
- Now picture a room – real or imagined. Notice all the details in the room, and see how welcoming it looks.
- Notice there is a comfortable chair in the room which is near a

fireplace – as close or as far away as you want to be from the fireplace.

- Settle comfortably into the chair and relax. Watch the fire, its beautiful colours and soothing sounds relaxing you. Imagine your gaze softening as you watch the flames dance.
- Now think of any concerns, worries or negative beliefs you have about your upcoming birth – or indeed anything. Feel them all held tightly inside your hand.
- Once you've gathered them all, open your hand and one by one, throw each concern into the fire. Let each one go and watch the flames increase briefly as they engulf and burn each concern.
- Take your time until you have let go of all that you want to let go of. Notice yourself feeling lighter and more at ease with each concern that has been released into the flames.
- When you are done, relax for a moment, enjoying feeling positive, light and free. Let these good feelings spread throughout your whole body and mind. And when you're ready you can slowly become more aware of the room, your surroundings and open your eyes – or drift off to sleep if appropriate.

You can also ask yourself the following questions:

- This concern I have – how likely is it to happen to me?
- What, if anything, might I be wrongly assuming about things?
- How might my thoughts and feelings be distorted – is this my truth, or is it someone else's story?
- What unreasonable demands am I placing on myself (to have the 'perfect' birth)?
- What, if anything, am I mistaken about? (This is why doing your research is so important)
- Is there anything I'm not thinking about logically?
- How true is my concern, objectively, as a percentage, and if it truly is on the cards, who can I talk to in order to gain some perspective on it all and ask questions?
- What can I do today to move away from or research my concerns so I am more positively focused?
- What would be a more helpful way of thinking about all of the above?

If you still feel, after honestly thinking about your fears, that they are very real for you, focus on listening to the fear release script/MP3 (you can find the script at the end of the book) until you start to feel a shift or change.

Read other hypnobirthing/positive birth books and saturate your brain with as many different sources of positive birth stories as possible. If at all possible, attend a hypnobirthing course in person.

If after all of this the fear feels still very intense, or you have a difficult past birth experience to work through, it may be useful to have some sessions with a qualified and experienced cognitive behavioural hypnotherapist, perhaps alongside a cognitive behavioural therapist (the latter you may be able to get referred to via your GP). Specialist referrals can also be done by your midwife.

Mindfulness

The following is a very brief outline of mindfulness. Mindfulness is a whole course and book in itself! I refer you to Jon Kabat-Zinn, founder of Mindfulness Based Stress Reduction (MBSR) for more in-depth information on mindfulness if it is something that interests you.

Kabat-Zinn has defined mindfulness meditation as 'the awareness that arises from paying attention, on purpose, in the present moment and non-judgmentally'. By focusing on the breath, the idea is to cultivate attention on the body and mind as it is moment to moment, and so help with pain, both physical and emotional.

Mindfulness is stepping back, and pausing between thoughts and reactions rather than engaging with them. Accepting that our thoughts are not fact, or our reality. It is paying attention in the present moment for as long as you are able to rather than raking over past events or imagining or worrying about future events. This is all harder than it sounds.

Mindfulness is taking time out for yourself and looking at things with an open mind so we can become less stuck in our ideas and opinions. This can be tricky, as of course we all have lots of opinions on everything – which is okay! It's more about becoming more aware of how judgemental we really are. We may notice how 'black and white' our thinking can be – but in a non-judgemental way. It helps us to be aware that we only see things through our own personal lens.

Mindfulness means accepting that things are the way they are, and not being caught up in things being a certain way (this is very useful for birth). This doesn't mean we don't do anything, or that we cannot try to change things, but rather we don't try to force change. If we don't accept things as they are we don't know where we stand, and if we don't know where we stand we can't take the first step to change things.

It's about trust – we trust our body will breathe for us and support us in every way. We don't think about our organs working or our ears hearing, we just take it for granted – until things go wrong. Our bodies can remind us that we are trustworthy and we can also learn to trust our mind and our ability to meet whatever comes our way.

Mindfulness is about patience – letting things unfold in their own way. When we are impatient we are always rushing things. Certain things can't be hurried – and childbirth is one of those things.

Mindfulness can help us to become aware of the many, many random thoughts that we have. Random thoughts are less easy to control, especially in difficult situations or when worrying about something that's playing on our mind – but you can control what happens next.

There is a lovely, short cognitive diffusion exercise (cognitive diffusion is a by-product of mindfulness) called 'Leaves on the Stream', which helps you to notice and become aware of and let go of random thoughts – whether positive or negative. We have a continuous flow of thoughts, many of which we are not even aware of and some of which we focus on to a very great extent! Leaves on the Stream helps you to allow thoughts to come and go without clinging on to them and struggling with them.

With cognitive fusion, we act as if thoughts are real and we respond as if our thoughts are all facts; this can have a physiological effect on our nervous system and provoke a stress fight or flight response. We get the same stress response from thoughts as we do from real events.

Cognitive diffusion is about detaching, taking a step back and allowing a pause between our thoughts and our reactions – to notice we are 'doing' thinking in the same way that we notice we are 'doing' other activities like brushing our teeth. 'I notice I am having a thought about X'. This helps us separate thoughts from reality, for example:

- I'm worried about giving birth
- I'm thinking I'm worried about giving birth
- I'm noticing I'm having a thought – I'm worried about giving birth

Thoughts – believe them, struggle with them or simply notice them. Our thoughts are just 'bubbles' coming to the surface – try seeing them as mere hypotheses rather than facts.

You can find the Leaves on the Stream script within the scripts section at the end of the book, and it is also available as an MP3.

How will practising mindfulness help during pregnancy and birth?

- It allows you to slow down and create space for yourself.
- Mental rest reduces stress, which is of great benefit for you and your baby.
- Your blood pressure and heart rate will lower when you're relaxed.
- It's important to block time off for yourself when you are pregnant and, at the very least, a few minutes of mindfulness practice a day is an easy way to help with this.
- It encourages you to pay attention to and appreciate your incredible, changing body.
- It helps you to become aware that thoughts are not facts.
- When in labour it will help you to accept how your birth unfolds – something we don't always have control over.
- It allows you to be present and to let go of any preconceived ideas of how your birth should be.
- It allows you to notice the rest time in between surges rather than worrying about the one you've just had or the next one on its way. This allows you to fully, mentally rest in between each surge.

Mindfulness is an excellent skill to use for life once your baby is here, and beyond.

The following three-minute breathing space mindfulness exercise is available as an MP3. Listening to it a few times may be useful until you are familiar with the process. Once it is familiar, you can use this calming, short exercise whenever you want to.

Three-minute breathing space

This popular mindfulness exercise has three parts. You can spend around a minute on each part, but it could be any length of time depending on what you want at that time, or how much time you have available.

Sit comfortably – though you can also do this exercise standing or lying down.

1. Expansive awareness

- Allow yourself to just take a gentle pause on life now. What can you hear and see around you? Are there any smells or other sensations?
- Close your eyes and become aware of your thoughts, feelings and the way your body feels.
- Notice what you are feeling at this moment, physically and emotionally. What do you notice about your posture and how your posture feels? Do you feel particularly comfortable in any way and if so where is this? Be curious about what thoughts you are aware of going through your mind at this moment. Can you place a little distance between yourself and your thoughts?
- Try and observe your thoughts non-judgementally and in a detached way rather than being caught up in them.

2. Narrowing into breathing

- Narrow your attention now to inside yourself and your own breathing.
- Bring your attention down to your breathing and the gentle rise and fall of your abdomen.
- You're not trying to change your breathing in any way, just simply being aware of it in an open way. It's usual for your attention to wander away from your breathing and if this happens, just notice where your attention has gone and then gently lead it back to your breathing again.

3. Expanding awareness

- Allow your conscious awareness to expand once again, from your abdomen and into your whole body. If you can, notice a feeling of breathing into your whole body. Become aware of your posture, your facial expression, sensations on the surface of the skin and from right inside your body. Just be fully aware now of any sensations in your body, just as they are. Enjoy the space around your body. Enjoy being here, right now, appreciating the present moment.
- See if you can be aware of a sense of wholeness and completeness in yourself, fully accepting and non-striving, okay to be just who you are at this moment. And just enjoy a moment of peace and stillness.

When you're ready, open your eyes and have a stretch.*

---

* Mindfulness exercise courtesy of UK College of Hypnosis and Hypnotherapy. **www. ukhypnosis.com**

Visualisation

Most people underestimate their ability to picture images – images don't need to be perfect or in sharp focus like a photograph in order to be good enough, nor do you need to see the whole scene in its entirety. For example, if you can give directions to the nearest train station or imagine showing someone around your home then you're able to visualise. Keeping it simple is fine.

Studies show that when you imagine something your brain and body respond much as they would if you experienced the real thing. Imagining an act can activate and strengthen parts of the brain involved in its real-life execution.

Visualisation works because neurons (which are cells that transmit information) in our brains interpret imagery as a real event. When we visualise an event or act, the neurons 'perform' the act (the 'act' in our case being a positive and calm birth experience). Visualisation is like a mental warm-up, conditioning your mind to recognise how it will act positively in response to your baby's birth (or whatever it is you are visualising).

Regular visualisation starts to create new neural pathways, which means our brain will create new learned behaviours, priming our body to act in a way consistent with our visualisation. All of this takes place without experiencing the physical activity.

A study in 2018 (the link is in the references section) suggested that imagination may be a more powerful tool than previously believed, and that we can use it to change the way we think about and experience things.

When you use visualisation, visualise in the first person, seeing any images through your own eyes rather than watching yourself as if on a screen. Start from the beginning (process visualisation) and imagine your birth journey, how you stay strong and breathe calmly through each surge, to the end where you're holding your baby in your arms (outcome visualisation) – you did it! It's important to use positive emotion when you're visualising your birth, so your thoughts are strong enough to leave an impression. For both types of visualisation it's good to bring as much detail in as possible, using all of the senses.

As already mentioned, the brain cannot tell the difference between a real or imagined event – just like when you get scared at a horror film or cry at a sad film – these aren't real events, but the brain interprets them as real. Repeatedly visualising your birth in a positive way means you're helping to wire your brain for a positive birth experience and therefore you're less likely to have fear arise.

So take time to regularly imagine how your birth will be. How smooth and calm it will be. Add as much detail as possible. This is a lovely thing to do before bed so that you fall asleep with your positive birth story in your head rather than a bad news story from scrolling through social media or a news app, or worrying about what you need to get done at work the next day.

Throughout the day keep an eye on and pay attention to how your mind wanders and what you choose to imagine. Spend time using your imagination for all the good, useful reasons.

Here are some suggestions you can use when using visualisation techniques to prepare for your baby's birth:

- Who will be there on the day? Picture them. What are they wearing, saying, doing?
- What will it smell like? Is there a scent you like that you will be bringing with you? Use the same scent that you used during your hypnobirthing practice as this will act as a trigger, reminding you of a time when you felt calm, confident and trusting of your body.
- What will the atmosphere be like? How dark, peaceful and calm will it be? Perhaps you will have battery-operated candles or fairy lights set up to create a spa-like zone.
- How will you feel when you are in labour? How relaxed, strong and calm?
- What can you hear – particular music? Encouraging words from your caregivers? One of the MP3s, or your partner's familiar voice?
- What can you feel – your partner massaging you or giving you a lovely bear hug? Or perhaps there is no touch, but you are feeling your deep calming breaths in.... and out.... Can you feel the soft material of your favourite pyjamas, or perhaps the warm water of the birthing pool?
- See yourself looking at your baby in your arms – you did it! How amazing and in awe will you feel? Feel the joy, the pride, the excitement and relief! Feel your baby's warm, soft skin and their weight in your arms.
- Add in as much precise detail as possible, involving all of your senses.

If you can, go and visit where you will be giving birth – look at the birth centre or the labour ward to further build up your imagery.

Affirmations

The idea of affirmations – which are statements said or written down repeatedly with emotion and confidence – is that when we repeat something over and over, it convinces our mind that it is true.

Affirmations can help to 'programme' your mind into believing what you are repeatedly stating or writing down – similar to how visualisation works.

When you say or write your affirmations, do so in the present tense, as if they are happening now, not in the future. Some examples are given below, though you can of course create your own, or find many more suggestions with a quick internet search. Even if you only find one you like, focus on that. Write or type it out and stick it up around your home on the wall, the fridge, or even the back of the toilet door! Anywhere you will notice it frequently and on a daily basis. It's all about repetition to embed the positivity firmly in your mind, so you start to change the way you think and feel about birth, replacing fear with confidence and trust.

You can also get really creative if this is your thing and create a birth vision board using pictures, quotes and affirmations. If you prefer to keep it simple then just write your affirmations on to post-it notes. Say them out loud and in your head.

There is a breathing and positive affirmations script at the end of the book, and an MP3 is available. Below are some affirmation suggestions:

I choose to feel good being me, I know I am capable.

I give birth easily and calmly.

My birth is smooth and comfortable.

I believe I can and so I will.

Each breath and surge (or contraction) brings my baby closer to me.

Women all over the world are giving birth with me.

Breathing deeply and slowly relaxes my muscles, making my labour comfortable.

My body knows how to birth my baby.

I am strong and I trust my body knows what to do.

I relax into each surge, maximising oxygen to me and my baby.

I keep gently active, I create space for my baby to be born swiftly and easily.

All is well.

Surges are powerful and strong, but they are not stronger than me because they are me.

I am using my surges to birth my baby.

I relax and let my body take over to birth my baby.

I am ready and looking forward to the birth of my baby.

I breathe in relaxation, I breathe out softness.

As labour progresses my relaxation deepens.

Whatever turn my birth takes, I remain calm and in control.

I am able to make decisions about my birth clearly and calmly.

The power of words

A woman in labour is an incredible force. I am continually amazed at a woman's power. Despite this, it doesn't take much to knock a woman's confidence when she is in the vulnerable state of giving birth – and many things can do this, words being one of them.

How information is relayed, and the choice of words used, can make a big difference. I use the word 'surge' (some prefer 'wave' or 'rush') instead of the word 'contraction' as it's a more pleasant way of describing the work of the uterus. A surge of energy or a wave in the sea will have a rhythm to it: it begins, builds, peaks and then peters out, just like a labour surge does.

You may also like to consider in advance not only how you feel about having internal examinations to establish (among other things) how dilated your cervix is, but also how you'd like this information delivered to you.

For example, would you like your partner to relay this information to you, or are you happy for the midwife to tell you? Remember that an examination only offers a snapshot of time, so although it may have taken you 'X' number of hours to get to say, 5cm dilated, this doesn't mean that it will take the same amount of time again to get to be fully dilated.

Rather than being told the numerical facts of how many centimetres dilated you are, perhaps you'd simply rather know whether or not you are progressing well.

To demonstrate the power of words, below are two different ways the same information can be conveyed:

Midwife 1: *'You're only about 4cm dilated, not quite halfway there yet.'*
Midwife 2: *'You are progressing beautifully, you're almost halfway there! You have so much confidence and calmness about you. Just keep taking one surge at a time and know that each surge is bringing you closer to meeting your baby. Before you know it your baby will be in your arms.'*

The author Rudyard Kipling once wrote: *'Words are, of course, the most powerful drug used by mankind'.* He was describing how a certain choice of words can change and influence how a person thinks and feels.

How do you want to receive information when in labour? Consider this carefully.

Creating positive cues/triggers and using post-hypnotic suggestions

We can create cues or triggers to help to establish a more resourceful state – one where we feel relaxed, strong, positive – or whatever state it is you want to feel. An example of a trigger could be when you hear a song and it takes you back to being at school, or you catch the smell of a perfume which reminds you of your best friend.

Repetition and mental association create a powerful link between a definite sensation e.g. pressing your thumb and forefinger together, and various emotional and psychological responses. This is further enhanced during hypnosis.

During hypnosis, once you're in a state of comfort, confidence or whatever the target state is, you are invited to link this with a physical gesture. This physical gesture creates a cue for positive feelings in the here and now, which can then be used to actively evoke the response you want during your labour or whenever needed. You can also use this technique to release negative feelings, or you can combine both, as required. It's just a way of using your memory.

You can also use a certain scent, such as lavender, to act as a cue or trigger. Each time you undertake any hypnobirthing or breathing practice, have your chosen scent to breathe in, to remind you that you are indeed prepared, confident and relaxed, and use this scent on the day. If possible, breathe this scent in while listening to your MP3s and at the end of the MP3, to 'lock in' and associate the scent with all the positive and relaxed feelings you will have.

Some scripts in this book include post-hypnotic suggestions. An example of a post-hypnotic suggestion is 'From now on, each and every time you feel anxious you give these feelings a colour which you can easily breathe out and release. And with each breath you feel calmer, stronger and more in control'. Post-hypnotic suggestions are very useful and are something you can apply quickly, helping you to call forth a positive way of behaving and acting when in the moment.

Post-hypnotic suggestion exercise using a physical cue

You would use this exercise in between surges, when your partner notices adrenalin or tension building – for example, they can see your breathing has started to become panicky or shallow, or you're breath-holding. Or perhaps there were interruptions in your quiet space or you had a powerful surge and are starting to lose your focus. You can use this exercise then as it's fast-acting.

As with everything, the idea is to practise this now so you know which body parts and words to use on the day. For example, if you know you always hold tension in your shoulders when stressed, you could focus on this body part.

Before you do this exercise think about what resourceful state you want to call upon – it could be a feeling of calmness, power and strength, being in control, or your body feeling soft and relaxed. You can also use your chosen resourceful state at the end of the MP3s when you are invited to 'lock in' all your good feelings with a physical gesture.

To practice antenatally

- Sit down with your partner (though in labour you would of course be in whatever position you are in)
- Birth partner uses a slower, quieter voice than usual, as with all the scripts
- Use the words 'When you feel/when I xxxxx (describe your action) you respond by xxxxx (describe what you want them to do)

1. Start by inviting the person to relax: 'Sit comfortably and close your eyes and take a long, slow breath in through your nose all the way down into your belly, then exhale through your mouth. Let all stress and tension be carried away on the out-breath. Repeat this three more times now (pause to allow for this).

   Now relax your facial muscles and allow your jaw to relax and open slightly, let your shoulders drop and your arms and hands rest comfortably, feel your back relax, your bottom and hips. Let your legs fall comfortably apart and feel your legs and feet becoming heavy and relaxed. Now breathe in slowly and breathe out slowly for a few breaths. Let your face relax... let your body relax... let your breathing relax.

2. Your partner can then insert the suggestion using your chosen resourceful state, e.g. 'When I place my hands on your shoulders you respond by breathing in, and on the out-breath releasing all tension/ letting that surge go/releasing all adrenalin/' or 'When I stroke my hand down your back you respond by allowing your whole body to sink into relaxation/to feel strong and in control', and so on.

3. Slight pause.

4. Your partner then places their hands on your shoulders, saying 'release all tension' or 'let that surge go' or strokes down your back saying 'sink into relaxation'.

5. You respond by taking the action suggested, such as releasing all tension.

6. Your partner repeats the suggestion again and then invites you to open your eyes when you are ready.

7. Keep the suggestions short, clear and simple.

During active labour, I'd suggest skipping stage 1 and instead just completing steps 2-6.

Pre-surge body scan

Sometimes women tense up as they feel the next surge starting, greeting it with a tight jaw, shoulders and body.

There is a script at the end of the book, the Top-to-Toe Tension Release, which will help you to practise this, but it is explained below.

Try to relax as soon as you feel the next surge starting to build. Greet it with a slow out-breath or sigh, and carry out a mental scan of your body from top to toe. Is your brow furrowed? Soften it and allow it to smooth out. Are your eyes scrunched up? Relax all the tiny muscles in and around them. Is your jaw clenched? Gently release it a little, allowing it to fully relax (some people find it useful to place the tip of their tongue behind their two front teeth as a reminder to slightly open and relax the jaw). Are your shoulders bunched up towards your ears? Drop them down to their natural relaxed state. Open and relax your fingers and palms.

Once you've practised it a little, this will take a split second to do, and releasing all tension as you feel the surge building allows your mind and body to be ready to take it on. You might like to imagine a wave or waterfall of relaxation starting at the top of your head and going all the way down to your toes, removing any tension as it passes through you, out and down into the ground. Remember, the surge will only last for around a minute.

If, while being aware of the power of the surge, you are able to make your whole body relaxed and limp, breathing deeply and gently, fear will not arise. Talk to your birth partner about where you have now noticed that you tend to hold tension in your body and ask them to remind you to relax those areas if they notice them tensing in labour. For example, if your shoulders are your natural area of tension, as your surge begins your birth partner can keep an eye out for this. They can then remind you to release and drop them down, perhaps gently pressing down on them or stroking, and using your trigger word such as 'relax', 'release', 'soften' or 'let go'.

Practising this in advance will make it easier for you to release tension at the start of each surge. It gives you a little plan of action you can repeat for each surge.

Remember, all you need to do is to handle and focus on one surge at a time.

Like all the techniques, this isn't something you do a few times and then expect it to work on the day. It's a skill that you are learning in order to be able to relax despite feeling the intensity of the surges, and like most skills, it takes practice and repetition before it feels like second nature.

Breathing

At the risk of sounding repetitive, using specific breathing techniques during labour and birth is the most important tool you have at your disposal. If you were to get one thing nailed, working effectively with your breath is that one thing. It's literally foundational for a calm and as-relaxed-as-possible birth. It is pretty much impossible to panic when you are breathing slowly and rhythmically. Tension and relaxation cannot exist in the same body at the same time – so let relaxation be your chosen state!

When a labouring woman is relaxed, her surges can do the job they are meant to do. This means that her uterine muscles work together as nature intended – the upper segment of the uterus works strongly and with each successive surge the muscle fibres of the upper segment become shorter and thicker (retraction) which in turn draws the weaker, thinner part of the lower uterus up. This dilates the cervix, gradually moving the baby downwards.

> *Researchers think that relaxation for pain relief may work by interrupting the transmission of pain signals to the brain, helping you focus on something positive, so giving you a positive source of distraction, stimulating the release of endorphins (your body's natural pain-relieving hormones), and reframing your thoughts to think of labour sensations as positive, productive and manageable....* *Relaxation techniques are safe to use and may have benefits such as reducing pain during early labour and reducing rates of other interventions such as epidurals.* Dekker, R: 2018. Relaxation for pain relief during labour

Conversely, tension in the mind and body is more likely to cause more pain, and will feed into the Fear-Pain-Tension cycle, increasing adrenalin and slowing labour down. The breathing you are now familiar with is the best way to help yourself. And not only that, it's a great life skill to be able to go within yourself and calm yourself quickly using just your breath.

Remember, the peak of the surge is only around 20-30 seconds long, which is 2-3 big, slow, deep breaths. By the time you are on the fourth/fifth breath the surge will be petering out. You can do anything for around 30 seconds.

Learning breathing techniques is not only for the labouring woman, but also the birth partner, who can benefit from using them to stay relaxed and calm on the day. Encourage your birth partner to practise as well. They are also very useful postnatally.

I invite you to reread Chapter 11 on breathing and try out the exercises at the end of that section. Try out the different visualisations even if you're not sure that's your thing – you never know what might be useful on the day. Carve 10 minutes out of your day for your breathing practice. I can guarantee that no woman ever looks back and says 'Oh, I did way too much breathing practice!', but many do say that they wish they'd done more. It needs to be second nature, so you are so well versed in it that it is effortless to slip into it.

Remember not to be disheartened if you find that you're not able to get your out-breath very long at first – this will improve with practise and repetition.

Tips for including your hypnobirthing practice in your everyday life

- Schedule it in. Literally set aside time. For example: on a Tuesday, Thursday and Sunday, for 10-15 minutes, do one of the couple's relaxations/scripts or some massage practice while dinner is cooking. If you tag it onto the end of the day chances are you'll be too tired and sleepy after dinner to do it or say 'We'll do it tomorrow instead'. And tomorrow will come... and go... with nothing achieved, again. So deliberately set time aside.
- Build the exercises in this chapter up slowly, then increase the frequency of your practice as you get closer to your due date. If you have plenty of time then doing some practice three times a week is great. If you are short of time or the due date is looming, then increase the practice. You'll never look back and say 'We did way too much practice, we were far too prepared!'
- Play your positive affirmations MP3 while you're getting ready for work, in the bath, preparing dinner, pottering about, and so on. Actively listen to them, adding emotion and feeling, repeating them out loud or in your head.

- Use the MP3s if you wake in the night unable to go to sleep. This is a better use of your time than tossing and turning and the relaxation elements may help you to nod off.
- Read some or all of this book and others together as a couple. How about reading or re-reading chapters out loud to one another as a way to share information and know that your birth partner has heard what you want them to hear?
- Watch a birth video once a week. Watching a positive birth video can be a powerful antidote to all the negative, dramatic rubbish we see on TV about birth.
- Try daily breathing and visualisation practice. It may be easy to breathe deeply and calmly now, but when in you are in advanced labour, if you have not done any breathing practice, it will be harder to relax on command.
- We have already talked about visualisation, but as a reminder, spend time visualising your birth with as much detail as possible. This is a lovely thing to do before you fall asleep at night or when sat waiting for something, such as in a traffic jam or when waiting for the train to work.
- Create a birth board with wedding photos/couple photos, scan photos, holiday photos, affirmations and positive birth quotes (all written in the present tense). If a birth board isn't your thing, then simply stick your positive affirmations and quotes all over your home on post-it notes. It might not sound like much, but noticing them, reading them and repeating them will make a difference. It's all about the repetition.
- Really go for it. You will not regret having put the effort in. It really makes all the difference when a couple/woman has done regular practice. You won't get a second chance to birth your baby so give it all you've got.

Suggestions for how to use your hypnobirthing when in labour

You've read this book, maybe completed a hypnobirthing course and focused on the all-important practice. Your baby is on the way now, so how should you use your hypnobirthing techniques? What do you do when?

The good thing about hypnobirthing is that there are no rules. You have a toolbox of techniques and are familiar with a variety of scripts to pick and choose from, plus the powerful tool of self-hypnosis. Some

MP3s/scripts you will likely prefer to others and find more relaxing and beneficial, so do what feels right for you.

Below are ideas on how you can use hypnobirthing for each stage of labour. Remember there are suggestions in Session 4 on other things to do in labour too.

Early labour

- You may wake in the night feeling your surges start. Put on your favourite MP3 or use self-hypnosis and try to go back to sleep.
- If it's daytime, curl up on the sofa, maybe use an eye mask and have your partner read out one of the scripts or listen to an MP3 – you may doze off, and at the very least you will be resting and conserving energy.
- Have your positive affirmations MP3 or one of the other MP3s playing in the background or on headphones. Their familiarity will be comforting to you.
- Stroking or light touch massage may feel good now.
- Try the birth ball.

Active labour

- Once things are in full flow you will find it useful to start focusing on your breathing.
- Massage may or may not be of interest.
- Words of encouragement from your partner in between surges can help. Let them know what affirmations you like.
- If of interest, continue to use the MP3s and scripts in whatever way works for you.
- Use the birth ball if you're finding it helpful.

Time to go in

- Earphones at the ready and MP3 on in the car/taxi if you want to really stay in the zone. If your partner can sit with you in the back all the better. Perhaps they could read one of the scripts out to you. Eye mask or sunglasses?
- Arrive in hospital and meet your midwife. Ask your partner in advance to ensure your birth preferences are read.

- Get all the lights down, listen to a whole script from your partner or put your favourite MP3 on. All of these things will ground you as you've listened and practised with them for so long during your pregnancy. Just hearing your partner with their familiar voice saying words you know so well will help to relax and calm you.
- Play the MP3s via a small speaker.
- Your breathing will be of great use now. Co-breathing may be useful too.

Transition

- Lots of encouragement from your partner and use the post-hypnotic suggestion exercises in between surges.

Time to meet your baby

- Most women find that they no longer want to focus on scripts or MP3s at this exciting and intense time. Keep those oxygen-fuelled breaths coming, sending your breath downwards to nudge your baby out. Consider your position and remember how the pelvis looked when a woman was flat on her back, how it leads to a restriction in space and how helpful gravity is.
- Postnatally you can continue to use the breathing and other techniques, as being able to relax at will is a fabulous skill to have learned. There is a postnatal script included at the end of the book.

All the scripts and affirmations in this book are available as MP3 downloads and the written versions are at the end of the book. Each MP3 is available with background music, and without. To access all the MP3s visit this link: www.baby-bumps.net/bookmp3s.

It can be lovely to have your partner read the scripts to you. If you like, they can include a physical cue such as an arm or hand stroke, or placing their hands on your bump, each time they read out the scripts. If they are consistent with this it will act as a trigger to remind you of feeling confidence and trust around birth. You can then use this on the day at any point in your labour either on its own or combined with your trigger word. Remember to include breathing in the scent of your choice each time too.

Final tips

Your role in hypnosis is to remain as physically comfortable and mentally receptive as possible. Keep thinking positively, and just imagine agreeing with the positive suggestions. You will only accept suggestions which you choose to accept. When listening to the MP3s or your partner reading out a script, imagine that any sounds from around the room or sensations in your body can simply cause you to go deeper into hypnosis.

It's okay if your mind wanders during hypnosis and relaxation, this is to be expected. Just patiently guide your attention back when you notice this happening.

Remember, don't worry if it feels a bit strange at first to have your partner read the scripts out. Eventually you'll get past this and find yourselves looking forward to this time together. The more you practise hypnosis, the better you will get at responding to the suggestions. Let go of any preconceptions from television shows or stage acts and just allow yourself to be open-minded.

Birth partners – when you read out a relaxation script, try and keep your voice soft and slow, with plenty of well-placed pauses.

You don't have to sit perfectly still throughout the MP3s/scripts, but the more you do, the less awareness you'll have of your body. Stillness means that you tend to have fewer distractions. When embarking on your practice, find a comfortable place where you will be undisturbed, sit upright and be attentive, ideally with your feet flat on the floor, and arms and legs uncrossed.

While it's great to relax, and this is a wonderful side effect of hypnosis, if you get so relaxed you can hardly move a muscle it is unlikely that you are going to be able to respond to suggestions (unless of course the suggestions being given and the purpose of the script was purely for relaxation!). If you can stay receptive, alert, attentive and focused you will find it much easier to achieve the outcome you want.

Remember, everyone can be hypnotised because everyone is able to change their beliefs and use their imagination. All you need to do is imagine you are agreeing with all the positive suggestions within the scripts and think and imagine along with it all. There's no need to try too hard or to worry about how well you are doing.

Positive birth stories

Below are a few positive birth stories covering different birth scenarios. All are from my clients, with their names removed for confidentiality. These birth stories, and many others, are shared with permission on my website **www.baby-bumps.net**. I include them here so you can see how hypnobirthing has worked for other real-life parents in many different ways.

Home birth

'I am sitting with my beautiful little four-week old baby daughter sleeping beside me and thought I would take this opportunity to write to you to say a huge thank you. We had such a wonderful birthing experience and couldn't have done it without the tools you provided us with during our hypnobirthing course. I gave birth in the water, at home and with no pain relief. The birth we had both wished for!

My first surge was at 6.30pm and actually took place while listening to a hypnobirthing track! My husband came home from work an hour or so later, at which point I was having a surge every 20 minutes or so. He set up a mattress in the living room with candles and calm music. He talked me through every surge, encouraging me to breathe and relax as we had practised. I used a TENS machine which really helped. He called the midwife at about 2am when the surges were longer and more frequent, and by the time she arrived I was 7cm dilated. The pool was now ready in our dining room (it took a long time to fill!) and my husband had used our fairy lights and music to create the same calm atmosphere. I was anxious about removing the TENS machine but the warm water felt wonderful.

Again, my husband was a huge support, physically and emotionally. Although I found it challenging to relax as I had done when we'd practised, I was certainly more relaxed than I would have been without our hypnobirthing mindsets. The music really helped as I associated this with the relaxation sessions I had been doing for the past few weeks.

For the next few hours my waters were being a bit stubborn and I decided to have them broken, after which things moved fairly quickly.

Our little girl was born at 9am and it was by far the best moment of our lives. I held her for 20 minutes in the water before my husband cut the cord and had some skin-to-skin time with her himself. The midwife stayed with us until lunchtime to make sure we were happy with feeding and left us snuggled up as a family to get to know our little baby girl. Four weeks later she still hasn't been to a hospital!

I would recommend hypnobirthing and if possible home birth so highly.'

Second-time mothers

'The birth was very different to P's... I managed to get through most of the contractions at home by breathing and focusing on music, as practised. Eventually she was born 20 minutes after I was measured being at 4cm dilated! We didn't even make it to the labour ward! But I feel happy and pleased with how things went, and proud of how I coped – only having gas and air!'

'So our little baby boy arrived on Wednesday. The hypnobirthing MP3s got me through, on repeat, in the early stages and into hospital where I was 6cm dilated with just an hour off delivery. Six hours in all so completely different to my first and I really do credit that with being in a completely different state of mind due to listening to the relaxations and practising hypnobirthing techniques every day.'

Second-time mother who was induced

'I gave birth to my daughter last Wednesday, and the hypnobirthing techniques were very successful. In the end I had to be induced at 40+12. I was warned that the pessary could cause pain, and to expect it to take at least 24 hours, so even though I started having contractions after a few hours, I was managing it so well with the breathing and visualisations that I didn't realise that I was actually in labour. As the contractions intensified I was so 'in the zone' that none of the staff realised I was in labour either, until my waters suddenly broke. Unfortunately, with all the fussing about what to do with me as the birthing centre and labour ward were full, not to mention a very intense and fast labour, I lost the flow in the final stage, so it wasn't a super calm birth, but it wasn't a nightmare ordeal like my first one and I didn't need any pain relief apart from my TENS machine and gas and air. After my waters broke it only took about an hour until my daughter was born – I didn't even leave the antenatal ward, though they did

*manage to wheel me into a private room at the last minute so I didn't
have to give birth in a corridor.*

*Incidentally, I think that one of the most useful things for me was
knowing how time passes much more quickly when you take slow
breaths, from that exercise where we counted how many breaths we
took in one minute – knowing that to be the case, it really helped make
the contractions more bearable in early labour.'*

Second-time mother whose baby arrived early

*'Our son came three weeks early and oh my did the hypnobirthing help!
I think it really preserved my energy for when I needed it. I also think
the midwives underestimated my progress as I was so silent. My actual
labour was about an hour!*

*Not just the birth, but I also think it helped with me calming down as
an individual. I started to cramp and saw my mucus plug three weeks
early, but still managed to present to the CEO, go shopping to get baby
bits, pack up my desk and go home to pack, all done while calm, happy
and no panic at all! I'm a very, very happy mum and really enjoyed
the newborn phase this time round. Also thanks for empowering me
to take off and throw away the belts they put around you which totally
restricted my thoughts and movements!'* [During a course we talk about
requesting intermittent monitoring, if appropriate.]

First-time mother who had an assisted birth

*'What a week! As you know my waters broke last Tuesday and then
my contractions began around 6pm on the Wednesday evening – I
went into hospital and was already 5cms dilated! Unfortunately I
had to stay on labour ward rather than go to the birthing centre as my
waters had gone over 24hrs previously, so the baby had to be monitored
throughout. I laboured without any pain relief and just used the
breathing techniques we had learned until 6.30am on Thursday when
it became apparent baby was unable to make her way out alone. Baby
was born with the help of a kiwi cap (and a spinal block!) at 7.53am on
30 April.*

*All of the staff commented on the relaxed nature of the labour and
how I coped with the contractions and baby was born with fantastic
Apgar scores despite the long labour. A helped massively during the
more intense contractions by reading out some of the scripts we had*

practised and it really focused me. Although we had to deviate from our birth plan I believe the hypnobirthing techniques we used were hugely beneficial when it came to making important decisions about the direction of the birth.'

First-time mother who had a fast active labour

'R is doing really well. It's so surreal being parents, we're loving it despite total sleep deprivation. My active labour ended up being 1 hour 25 minutes and I had her in the pool at the birth centre – only just. She came out in her sac so her head appeared like a little astronaut. She was 10 days overdue and was 7lb 3oz and it was a totally natural birth.

I had contractions from 1am at home, was in hospital at 4.30 and told I was 1cm. My contractions were regular every three to four minutes from the get-go so they told us to go for a walk for an hour. When I went back at about 6am, I was still 1cm dilated, so was sent across to the labour ward. Things must have progressed rapidly there, because pretty soon I was feeling an incredibly strong urge to push. A midwife measured me and said I was fully dilated and ready to push, so they whizzed me back to the birth unit, where I had to get into the pool straight away. Two pushes later she was born.

R was brilliant reminding me of the breathing techniques and remaining calm when the surges were at their most intense. The visualisations kept me very focused and confirmed to me the power of the mind-body connection. We were the talk of the birth unit as to how quickly everything happened. So delighted to have had such a positive experience and he is such content little baby.'

First-time mother – waterbirth

'Our son was born on 1 February weighing 7lb 8oz in the midwife-led unit. The techniques for breathing and relaxation, along with the use of water and counter-pressure, all allowed me to stick to our birth plan and have a drug-free delivery. I definitely couldn't have done it without P's support and hypnobirthing had absolutely prepared him for every stage of the labour – he was my advocate, cheerleader and guide throughout. Hypnobirthing armed us with the information we needed to make choices that helped us bring our son safely and naturally into the world.'

First-time mother and informed decision-making

'S was born 13 days late. From day one past my due date inductions were proposed to me. I declined to have a sweep at day one past my due date but after a week I did have one as I had been experiencing Braxton Hicks and also on examination I had begun to dilate, therefore things were already on the move. I had a second sweep at 10 days past my due date and at 12 days went to discuss my options with a consultant.

The consultant examined me and I was 2.5cm dilated by this point and I could feel S was much lower down, I was also experiencing stronger Braxton Hicks. Incidentally they found my fluid levels were slightly low and so the doctor advised I was admitted there and then to have my waters broken in theatre. I sought a second opinion about this and spoke with two senior midwives. I was advised that my fluid levels could have been low for a while and they weren't dangerously low.

I went against the doctor's advice, this was quite scary as I had to sign a consent form to self-discharge. I went into labour naturally that night and gave birth naturally in the midwife-led unit. I used the birthing pool and shower along with relaxation techniques and breathing control throughout the second stage of labour.

Hypnobirthing gave me the confidence and the knowledge to question the health professionals' advice and plans to induce me. I'm so glad I did as I managed a natural birth, and during monitoring S's heart rate was always normal so I feel that she entered the world in the best way possible and was not distressed.'

First-time mother

'My waters went on Thursday as I was walking up the stairs in the hospital to go have a blood pressure check! I wasn't having contractions so they booked me in for an induction the next morning.

So I went home and walked loads, went and had labour reflexology, and then thought I best just sleep! The next morning I was having gentle period-like cramps but they told me to come in anyway. I went in and at about 10.30am they put me in the induction ward.

The midwife came to give me the pessary and then said she couldn't as I was already 3cm. I said to her I was getting period pains so she decided to leave me to it for a while. Anyway out of nowhere it felt like they went from period pains to full-on contractions. They seemed to last minimum 90 seconds and then the gap between them was getting shorter and shorter. I wasn't being checked on as I think as a first-time mum they thought I'd be there for ages. Suddenly there was no let up between contractions and I thought if that wasn't transition I really needed drugs!! (I did have gas and air but it made me feel sick I couldn't use it) so I literally screamed the place down for a midwife — she came and examined me and I was 9cm.

I just knew I had to get out of the ward and into a delivery room (poor people who were in there with me! I think I panicked as nobody was around to check on me hence the screaming for a midwife!) I am laughing now because they kept on about being high risk and constant monitoring! So anyway at 5.35pm our little boy made an appearance! He weighed 6lb 2oz and was 53cm long. Midwives in delivery suite were amazing! I think I'd lost the plot by time I got into the delivery suite and was being a bit of a nightmare then! But once I got in I didn't panic at all during the pushing stage even when he got a little stuck and it took a bit longer – I think all the hypnobirthing helped with that – no tears or episiotomy thank goodness!

Funny thing is I so wanted to be able to move around and all I could do to get comfortable was lie down in the end!! I tried kneeling and standing for birth but I found lying down the best! Funny how you think one thing but another thing actually happens! Glad to be home now and working out a newborn! He's so cute!'

First-time mother with short hospital time

'We had our baby on Saturday 21 February at 5.39 pm and he weighed in at 7lb 5oz with no complications. He arrived one day before his due date.

We think the hypnobirthing really helped us. I started having mild contractions around 8pm on the Friday night but I managed to sleep through parts of the night, we spent the morning and early afternoon at home as the contractions had not reached a regular pattern, but by early afternoon they started getting quicker albeit I would have a couple of contractions 2-3 minutes apart and then might have a gap of 8-10 minutes and they were varying in length from 30 seconds to around a minute. By the time we reached the hospital at 4pm I was 7-8 cm dilated. We had half an hour on the labour ward (for an unknown reason the birth centre was closed) using some gas and air, by which point I was fully dilated and baby was born naturally 40 minutes later. We credit the short time in hospital to the preparation we did with the hypnobirthing.'

End-of-session summary

You've now learned about the power of the mind and the benefits of hypnobirthing. I invite you to try out all the elements within the chapter, for example:

- Have a listen to all of the MP3s and see which ones you like. Carve out 10-15 minutes a day to do some practice, which could be listening to an MP3 or some breathing, and ideally both!
- Think about what affirmations you will use and put these up around your house.
- Watch some hypnobirthing births on YouTube.
- Spend time visualising your birth before you go to bed.

"

Let's talk about pain manage-ment, assisted birth and healing

"

In the sixth session we talk about:

- All the different pain management options from epidural to water birth to using a TENS machine. What are their pros and their cons and how and when do you access them?

- Monitoring your baby – when may this be offered to you and what is involved?

- Assisted birth – what does this mean?

- Lastly, we'll cover stitches, healing and perineal massage.

Chapter fourteen

Pain management options

→ When it comes to pain management of course there is no 'one size fits all', and while some women are very focused on utilising the incredible tools they already have within themselves, others may have this in mind, but also want to explore medical options - or their initial preferences change during the course of their labour.

You have every right to change your mind during labour and opt for pain management if that is something you feel you need.

In this chapter we will look at the options available, so you are able to make an informed decision when the time comes. Some methods have already been covered, but a recap is offered in this chapter.

Hypnobirthing

Hypnobirthing (see Chapter 14) is a popular and effective method that uses deep relaxation, breathing techniques, visualisations, affirmations, **149** mindset overhaul and fear-release techniques to manage labour. Birth partners are very much involved from the outset and have a clear role in assisting their partner. Time is spent before the birth practising the techniques and working on releasing any fears.

Pros
- Women and partners feel empowered.
- Birth partners are very much involved.
- Often no pain relief medication is needed.
- Women are informed and educated about how their body works in labour.
- Women report feeling calm and in control whatever turn their birth takes.
- No side-effects for mother or baby – babies benefit from the increased oxygen from the constant deep breathing.

Cons
- There is a cost to do a course or to buy any book/s and MP3s.
- You need to practise in advance (which is very pleasant to do!).
- Some women find it only helps up to a certain point in their labour.

Breathing techniques

I know we've talked about this a lot already, but the importance of using breathing techniques cannot be underestimated. Deep, slow breathing is calming and brings valuable oxygen and a good blood flow to both mother and baby. Partners can be involved and can assist by using co-breathing if the mother starts to become panicked. Relaxed breathing has many benefits. Using breathing techniques will keep you relaxed. Tension and relaxation cannot exist in the same body at the same time. If you decide you would like medical pain relief, breathing techniques will still be of use for you and your baby.

Pros
- Free
- It increases blood and oxygen flow to mother and baby.
- Birth partners can be involved.
- It instantly reduces stress and tension.

- It gives you great focus.
- It increases birth hormones like oxytocin and endorphins, which help you feel calm and relaxed and in turn makes your surges more efficient.
- No side-effects for mother or baby; both will benefit from relaxed breathing.

Cons

- It takes time and effort to practise the breathing techniques (which is well worth it).
- Some women find breathing techniques only get them so far before they want additional methods.

Massage

Touch is comforting for most, although some women prefer not to be touched during labour. Touch can vary and includes gentle stroking, holding, firmer stroking, foot massage, hand massage and deep massage using palms or knuckles and counter-pressure. Usually the firmer massage is welcomed in the latter stages of labour. Touch may help a woman feel safe and secure and increases the production of the hormone oxytocin. If you want to, you can use certain essential oils diluted in a carrier oil.

Pros

- Provides comfort.
- Increases oxytocin and endorphin production.
- Reduces cortisol (stress hormone) levels.
- Can shorten the first stage of labour and decreases complications related to a prolonged labour.
- Improves the labour process.
- Birth partners are involved.
- No side-effects for mother or baby.

Cons

- Some women do not want to be touched in labour.
- It takes practice (I'm not sure this is a con though!)

Active birth (positions and movement)

Active birth is when a woman follows her body's lead and moves accordingly, rather than being on the bed, on her back, which makes surges slower and more uncomfortable. A woman's movement and position should not be restricted or dictated.

There are numerous studies on the benefits of using movement in labour. The Royal College of Obstetricians & Gynaecologists (RCOG) says that women should be allowed to make informed choices about which position they want to give birth in. NICE recommends that women should not be encouraged to lie flat or semi-flat, particularly in the second stage.

When a woman is supine (on her back), blood supply to the uterus and placenta is restricted due to the weight of the uterus pressing on certain blood vessels. Her blood pressure can also drop in this position. Being upright increases the pelvic capacity by up to a third, helping the baby move down as well as making the mother feel more comfortable.

Pros

- Movement and changing position are a good distraction and provide a focus.
- When you follow your instinctive urge to move it may encourage your baby into a good position and will make things feel more manageable.
- UFO (upright forward open) positions create more room in the pelvis for the baby.
- Being active may reduce the chance of needing a caesarean birth.

Cons

- You may feel tired, in which case you can lie on your left side to rest for a while. You can also give birth while side-lying.

Continuous support

There is much evidence of the benefits of a woman having a familiar, constant and calming birth partner present. This is why a home birth can be such a great option, as you may well have met your midwife several times in advance of the birth.

Emotional support boosts you and helps you feel supported and confident. Some women or couples decide to hire a doula for this very reason and doulas have been shown to reduce the need for pharmacological pain relief.

If your birth partner is someone who is likely to panic or they feel very anxious and are concerned about how best they can support you, hiring a doula or having a second birth partner available will be beneficial. When someone is nervous or frightened they will be pumping out adrenalin into the room, making it harder for you to relax and focus inward.

Water birth

If you've had a straightforward pregnancy you may like to use water during your labour, and this can include getting into a shower, a bath or a specially-designed birth pool, which is either plumbed in or inflated. If you are planning a home birth you will need to make arrangements to hire or buy one. Some home birth teams have pools available to borrow or hire. If your pregnancy has not been straightforward it's still worth asking in advance if you can use the pool as it may still be an option.

You can get in and out of the pool and enjoy the soothing benefits of being immersed in water whenever you like, as there is no evidence that getting in at a certain time is more beneficial than at other times. Some women prefer to wait until they are around halfway through their labour and get into the pool when they feel the surges are very intense. You can have all of your labour in the pool, or part of it. If you find your labour slows while in the water you may like to get out, walk about, empty your bladder and then get back in.

You can wear a tankini or bikini if you'd rather not take all of your clothes off. Sometimes birth partners get in the pool too to offer closer support.

Make sure you stay well hydrated.

If you are having a managed third stage (delivery of the placenta) you will need to get out of the pool for this; otherwise you can ask about staying in the pool until the placenta comes away. However, gravity can help with the third stage and in an emergency situation it is easier to help a woman when she is out of the pool, so your midwife may ask if you are happy to get out of the pool for this part of your labour.

It's normal for women to open their bowels in labour – the midwife will take care of this quickly should this happen when you are in the pool – and you probably won't even be aware of it.

Pros

- Enhances a feeling of privacy as you are immersed in the water.
- The buoyancy of the water allows for greater ease of movement. A lunge position is good for using in the pool.
- You can use gas and air in the pool.
- If you don't like it you can just get out.
- Someone will need to be with you at all times (midwife or birth partner) as you cannot be left alone in the pool.
- You and your baby will be regularly monitored in the same way throughout your labour as if you were on dry land.
- Research shows that there is less need for an epidural.
- You can use the sides of the pool to lean on.
- If you want to, you can slowly bring your baby to the surface once they are born – your midwife will guide you on how to do this, or she can do this for you if you prefer.
- While of course we can't speak for the baby, some believe it's a more gentle transition from womb to world when a baby is born in the water.
- There is no more risk of infection in the pool than there is for a woman giving birth on dry land.
- A water birth may shorten the first stage of labour.

Cons

- A pool may not be available when you want it – but you can use the shower you will likely have in your room, leaning forward on the wall with the water cascading down your back.
- The pool cannot be used if you need to be closely monitored or if you have had recent opiates (pain-relieving drugs).
- If a problem is suspected for you or your baby you will be asked to get out.
- If you decide you want an epidural or opiates you will need to get out of the pool.

- You cannot use a TENS machine in the pool.
- A water birth may not be recommended if you have had a more complex pregnancy – but it is still worth asking if you can use the pool if this is something you feel strongly about.

Gas and air (Entonox)

Gas and air (also known as laughing gas) is a mix of 50 percent oxygen and 50 percent nitrous oxide. In the UK it is available at home births and also in all birth centre and hospital settings. You inhale the gas through a mouthpiece until you start to feel a little lightheaded. It takes the edge off the surges and can make you feel giggly.

It takes about 15 to 20 seconds of breathing before you feel the benefits and it can take up to two or three minutes to get the full effect. It takes a bit of practice to get into the swing of it, so allow yourself time for this. To help get your rhythm, try taking 2-3 deep breaths of the gas and air at the very start of the surge – this should see you through that surge.

Pros

- It can encourage deep breathing and increased oxygen flow.
- In the UK it is readily available everywhere – home birth, midwife-led unit and labour ward.
- You can have it at any point during your labour, but it's great to use it once your labour is established when you may better feel its benefits.
- It is short-lasting, so if you do not like the effects they wear off in a few seconds once you stop using it.
- It won't negatively affect the baby and the increased oxygen may be beneficial.
- You are in control of how and when you use it.
- You can still move around while using it.
- You can use it in the birth pool. Your partner can help you by holding it in between surges so the mouthpiece doesn't fall into the water.
- You can use it alongside other pain relief such as a TENS machine or opiates.
- No additional monitoring is required for mother or baby.
- It won't impact the progression of your labour.

Cons

- The effects are mild – but this may be all you need!
- It's not recommended to use for long periods, so it may not be recommended if you are in very early labour since this can last many hours – or even days.
- While you can still move around, you will be a bit restricted due to holding onto the mouthpiece.
- Some women feel drowsy or nauseous and some are sick. Try to only breathe the gas and air during surges to help with this. Having regular sips of water and applying lip balm can help to manage a dry mouth.
- It can take a bit of getting used to in order to get the timing right so that the gas and air is most effective at the peak of the surge.

TENS machine

A TENS (Transcutaneous Electrical Nerve Stimulation) machine for labour is a small handheld device, about the size of a mobile phone, with four sticky pads, which you attach to your skin on either side of your spine. The device can be clipped on to your clothing if you prefer not to hold it. It delivers gentle, safe electrical current through the wires/pads, which give a tingly, pins-and-needles-type sensation. The electrical pulses pass through your skin and into the muscle/tissue.

Usually you start on the lowest level and work your way up by turning the dial bit by bit as labour progresses. Some machines have a boost button which can be pressed at the peak of a surge, but remember to turn this off afterwards so you feel the benefit next time.

There is only limited evidence on the effectiveness of TENS machines for reducing pain in labour. It is not known exactly how they work.

It is likely that they help by a combination of the following:

- It may change the way in which you perceive your discomfort in labour.
- When you use TENS at a low-intensity level, it may be working through 'gate control theory'. It's thought that only a certain amount of stimuli can get through to the brain, and if you're using a TENS machine you're already flooding the brain with a sensory buzzing feeling. Perhaps this then means you feel the surges less strongly.
- When you turn the TENS machine up or use the boost button the

intensity may cause a little discomfort, triggering your body to release endorphins.

- They give a feeling of control and offer distraction.

Usually hospitals and birth centres do not provide TENS machines, so it is up to you to hire or buy one. Not all TENS machines are suitable for labour, so make sure you hire or buy a maternity TENS machine.

It is best to set up the TENS machine when you are in early labour rather than established labour when your surges are strong. It can take a while for it to take effect, so try it for an hour or so before you decide whether or not it is working for you.

Pros

- As it is drug-free, a TENS machine will not negatively affect your labour or your baby.
- Other options will still be open to you (apart from a water birth – unless you remove the pads/machine!).
- If you do not like the sensation you can just turn the machine off and remove the pads.
- It can provide distraction and a feeling of control.
- You can move freely.
- You purchase a TENS machine, or hire (it costs around £25–35 for six weeks of hire) or borrow one, and can set it up yourself (your birth partner will need to place the pads in the right place on your back) without the need for a midwife or doctor.

Cons

- The pads can lose their stickiness, but a drop of water on them can help if this happens, or you can buy some spares. If you have sensitive skin ask if hypoallergenic pads are available.
- You cannot use the birth pool/shower/bath with the machine on.
- Your partner will not be able to massage your lower back.
- Do not use a TENS machine if you have a pacemaker, before you are in labour, before 37 weeks unless under medical supervision, or if you have epilepsy.
- If you do decide to use it in labour, pack spare batteries.
- Some women say they find using a TENS machine means they are

waiting for the next surge so they can press buttons, rather than staying in their zone.

Opioid drugs such as pethidine and diamorphine

Opioid painkillers are medicines with effects similar to morphine. They are usually given as an injection in the thigh and, as they can often make a woman feel sick, an anti-sickness drug is normally given at the same time which unfortunately isn't always effective.

Opiates can be given in differing doses. If you are very sensitive to drugs or are of a slight build, you may want to ask about starting on a lower dose. Doses can be repeated several times if required.

It takes around 20–30 minutes before the effects are felt. It's recommended to have opiates during the first stage of your labour. If your midwife thinks you are close to giving birth she won't offer you pethidine as it can make the baby drowsy and may affect their breathing.

Pros

- Some women find opiates help them relax and get some sleep, particularly if they have had a long first stage of labour and they are very tired.
- A midwife can administer pethidine and sometimes diamorphine so there is no need to wait for a doctor should you want this.
- It produces a sedation effect that can be helpful for some women who may be feeling very anxious.
- If you are in established labour it appears not to slow things down.
- It may postpone or prevent a woman from having an epidural if this is something she would prefer to avoid for reasons personal to her.

Cons

- Some people do not like the effects of opiates and it takes several hours for the effects to wear off.
- Women may feel some of these sensations: dizzy, drowsy, spaced out, detached and sedated – making labour harder to cope with.
- Opiates can make some women feel sick and vomit despite the anti-sickness drug.

- Pethidine only gives limited pain relief.
- A third of women who use pethidine find it unpleasant and the side-effects may make you feel less in control of your labour.
- Pethidine can make you feel drowsy and can slow your breathing so you may need oxygen through a mask to help with this.
- Diamorphine can make labour longer.
- All opiates cross the placenta and on occasion the baby may be slower to initiate breathing straight after birth if it is given close to giving birth.
- Opiates may make breastfeeding your baby less straightforward. Ask your midwife for help.
- If the drug is given close to the baby's birth it will take the baby several days to work it out of their system.
- It is likely that you will not be able to use the birth pool until the effects have worn off, although timings around this vary between hospital Trusts.

Epidural

Epidurals are around 90 percent effective in removing all pain and most of the feeling from around the waist down. It is a local anaesthetic injected into the epidural space between the vertebrae of the lower back and requires an anaesthetist to set it up.

You will be given a local anaesthetic in your back so you won't feel the epidural being inserted, though you will feel some pressure as this takes place. Occasionally it may not work and will need to be adjusted or taken out and reinserted.

An anaesthetist may not be available right away and you may have to wait for them. It takes around 20 minutes to insert an epidural and 20 minutes for the first test dose to take effect, which may be worth bearing in mind.

Having an epidural will mean continuous monitoring of the baby's heart rate and careful monitoring of the mother.

If a woman arrives in hospital and she is very tired, perhaps because she has had several days of on-off labour, she can ask about the possibility of having the epidural set up so that it enables her to get a few hours of unbroken sleep.

If a woman is keen to try to get into an upright position while she has an epidural she can request that the bed's position gets adjusted from being horizontal to being upright, like a dentist's chair. She could then position her legs/knees wide, with the support of pillows if needed, leaning forward with each surge.

She can also request that she is informed when she is reaching the end of the first stage of labour so that she doesn't receive or give herself any more top-ups. This can then mean that the effects of the epidural will fade away so she can feel to push and will possibly be able to adopt an all fours or kneeling position to give birth in, maximising all the space in her pelvis and utilising the force of gravity to help her baby be born.

Pros

- It gives total pain relief in most cases.
- Once it is set up it does not require an anaesthetist to top it up – a midwife can do this or you can self-administer a top-up via an epidural pump if this option is available.
- You will remain clearheaded.
- Some women are able to sleep and rest for a while as there is no (or very little) sensation felt, even though you may be aware of your surges.
- If the dose is low you may be able to move around on the bed and get into more upright positions – the peanut ball we talked about would be good to use.
- If you need to have a caesarean the epidural can be topped up for this purpose.
- In general, epidurals do not affect your baby.

Cons

- Around 10 percent of women only experience partial pain relief.
- If you are in the birth centre and you want an epidural you'll need to move to the labour ward and a room may not always be immediately available.
- You need to keep as still as you can when having an epidural or spinal, which is not always easy if the surges are very closely spaced.
- The sensations of birth encourage a woman to move about, which helps her baby get into a good position. With an epidural you will not

be able to move around completely freely, which may slow your labour down.

- It takes about 40 minutes before you feel the effects.
- There is an increased chance of needing forceps or suction (ventouse), particularly if there have been repeated top-ups.
- You may not have normal sensation when you need to empty your bladder so a catheter will likely be inserted to keep the bladder empty.
- You may need to be given drugs to augment your labour.
- There is a chance of lowered blood pressure, so you need an intravenous infusion (drip). This drip may be used for other reasons, such as to give medication to speed your labour up or if you are being sick.
- You may develop itching or a raised temperature (fever).
- The baby needs to be monitored closely with electronic foetal monitoring. This type of monitoring is associated with a higher rate of caesarean births.
- Usually a woman will be lying down after an epidural, so the powerful effects of gravity are not utilised. You can ask your midwife for help with moving onto your side or sitting more upright if you wish to – some hospital beds can be positioned in an upright chair position. Ask if there is a peanut ball to help with opening of the pelvis, or use pillows to help with this.
- Repeated top-ups may cause temporary leg weakness.
- It is currently not recommended that you eat after an epidural has been set up.
- Second stage will be longer and you are more likely to require synthetic oxytocin to speed this up.
- Some women experience a severe headache (uncommon) that can last for days or weeks if not treated. If you develop a headache talk to your midwife or anaesthetist.
- The epidural site may be sore for a few days after birth. Epidurals do not cause backache – though backache is common after pregnancy.

In some situations a spinal, which is a one-off injection into the small of the back, is given as this has a much quicker effect (5–10 minutes), though this is usually reserved for caesarean births and sometimes assisted births. With a spinal you are less likely to need a catheter for as long as you would with an epidural. Spinals last between 1–2 hours, depending on the dose given. They can't be topped up and are rarely given more than once. It takes around four hours, or maybe a bit longer, for it to wear off, and feeling itchy and tingly afterwards is normal.

Chapter fifteen

Monitoring

$\rightarrow$ Labour can sometimes be stressful for a baby – a strong, healthy baby can cope well with this, but if a baby is unwell or hasn't grown well it may be harder for them and it may be suggested that they are monitored continually. This is called electronic foetal monitoring (EFM). Your midwife may also use the term continuous cardiotocography (CTG) monitoring. EFM is only available on the labour ward, so not at home or at the birth centre.

NICE recommends intermittent monitoring for low-risk labours. This is used at a home birth and in birth centres and the midwife will listen in to your baby's heartbeat every 15 minutes in active labour. Intermittent monitoring is also used on labour wards unless mother or baby show signs of not coping well, or there is a medical intervention in the labour.

When might continuous EFM be recommended? Some examples are:

- For multiple pregnancy and breech position.
- If a mother has high blood pressure.

163

- If a mother has diabetes.
- When the waters have been released for over 24 hours – and broke before surges started.
- There is concern that the baby's birth is restricted.
- The waters have lots of meconium in them. Meconium is the baby's first poo and can sometimes indicate the baby is distressed.
- Raised maternal temperature, which may be pointing to an infection.
- Abnormal vaginal bleeding.
- If a mother has an epidural, has had her labour induced or has had her labour speeded up using synthetic oxytocin
- If a woman's labour becomes prolonged.

You may choose to decline continuous EFM after discussing it with your caregivers, or you may feel after your questions have been answered fully that you are happy to have it.

When you have continuous EFM, with the use of belts, one sensor is placed on your bump to measure your surges and another one is placed to measure your baby's heart rate. This information is relayed onto a print-out in the form of a graph and helps the midwife to be able to see how your baby is coping with the surges.

EFM can make movement more difficult and you may be told you need to stay still on the bed to be monitored – but you don't have to. You can still be active, but it may help if your partner holds on to the baby's heart rate sensor during a surge to try to stop the reading being lost as you move about. Perhaps you can ask for an additional stretchy belt (which holds the sensors on you) to go on top of the other one, so you double up with belts. This may hold the sensor more firmly when you move about. You can have the monitoring set up while you are on the birth ball so you can remain as active as possible throughout your labour.

If you need to be monitored continually, ask if telemetry is available – this is wireless monitoring that will not interfere with your movement.

EFM readings are not always accurately interpreted, and so your care should not be based just on the readings. Other things should be taken into consideration such as your baby's movements, how you are feeling, and other signs that may be pointing to complications.

Intermittent monitoring

This is done using a handheld device such as a Pinard stethoscope or Sonicaid. Your midwife will find the right area on your abdomen and listen to the baby's heartbeat for at least a minute every 15 minutes in active labour and every five minutes during the second stage. It doesn't usually affect movement or position. This is what will be used at a home birth, and if your midwife suspects there are any issues with the baby's heartbeat they will swiftly arrange transfer into hospital and your baby will be monitored more closely.

During a water birth your midwife can use a waterproof Sonicaid so you won't need to get out of the pool or lift your bump out of the water for her to listen in.

Foetal scalp electrode

This is a small clip which is placed on your baby's head to monitor their heartbeat. It can be used alongside other monitoring and may give a more accurate reading. This can only be set up if a woman's waters have released.

Foetal blood sampling

If the doctor would like to assess how much oxygen is in the baby's blood so they can tell how well they are coping with labour they may talk to you about foetal blood sampling. During this procedure a local anaesthetic is applied to your baby's head and, using a rod with a tiny blade, a small blood sample is taken from your baby's head.

While continuous monitoring definitely has its place, it can have some downsides and routine use of it is not recommended. As well as restricting a woman's mobility, and therefore her ability to cope with her labour well, it has been linked to an increased number of interventions in labour, including caesareans and assisted births.

NICE states *'Cardiotocography is not appropriate in the initial assessment of women at low risk of complications who are in labour. This is because it may lead to unnecessary interventions and does not provide any benefit to the baby.'*

Chapter sixteen

Assisted birth, stitches and healing

→ Forceps and ventouse are instruments that are used to help a woman birth her baby and when they are used it is called an assisted birth or instrumental birth. Forceps are used to turn a baby who isn't progressing down because they're in an awkward position. Ventouse is used if the labour is not progressing because the mother cannot push strongly enough for some reason (exhaustion, very long labour, epidural, etc).

Having an epidural and induction of labour makes an assisted birth more likely.

Having continuous support from someone you trust can reduce the chance of an assisted birth, as does being upright in labour and avoiding lying on your back to give birth.

If an assisted birth is being suggested, you may like to ask if it is okay to have a little time, even a few minutes, alone with your partner to get your head around it all. Of course if it is a true emergency it will be obvious and that's a different situation, but if not, a few moments alone may, for example, give you chance to perhaps change your position,

167

galvanise some energy, or to mentally process the change in plan.

Before an assisted birth a woman will have either an injection to numb the perineum, or a spinal – or she may already have an epidural in place. With her consent she will be examined internally and her abdomen will be examined. Her bladder will be emptied using a catheter. She will likely need to sit with her legs supported in stirrups. She may need an episiotomy (a surgical cut to the perineum) in order to have an assisted birth or if the baby needs to be born quickly. Any tears or episiotomies are repaired with dissolvable stitches and recovery usually goes well.

Sometimes a woman may have the procedure in theatre, and if the doctor is not reassured that the baby will be born safely by instrumental delivery, a caesarean birth may need to take place.

Forceps come in two halves. They carefully cradle the baby's head in the birth canal and, when the woman has a surge, she pushes and the doctor pulls at the same time, to help the baby out.

A ventouse is a small cap that is sometimes attached to a suction pump. The small cap fits onto the baby's head and stays attached with suction. The ventouse is then pulled to help the baby be born as the mother pushes.

It's quite usual for a paediatrician to be present in the room during an instrumental birth, so don't worry if you notice this. Sometimes the baby's head may be bruised, cut or misshapen following an assisted birth, but healing is usually straightforward.

Verbal consent is required before an assisted birth. It should always be explained to you why an intervention needs to take place.

Active management of the third stage is recommended after an instrumental birth.

Healing after a tear or an episiotomy

- Bathing in warm water and/or using a Valley cushion (a specially designed inflatable cushion to make sitting down more comfortable) may help you. You can hire Valley cushions – a quick internet search will bring this up. Some chemists stock them.
- Regular painkillers can help ease discomfort – your midwife will be able to advise which are safe to take if you are breastfeeding.
- Change your maternity pad regularly, washing your hands before and after.

- Keep an eye on your wound and let a midwife know if you have any red, swollen skin, pain that doesn't go away or any unusual smell. A woman should always have her stitches checked 24 hours after they've been done and, where relevant, before she leaves the hospital. They should also be checked on day five and day 10 or 14. If you find you're still very uncomfortable after these checks, speak with your midwife, health visitor or GP and don't suffer in silence. It could be that you have an infection which will make things more painful and slower to heal.

You might want to try the following suggestions during the healing period as well:

- You can pour warm water over your perineum while you wee if you are concerned about a stinging sensation – or wee in the shower or just before you get out of the bath. Try leaning forward when emptying your bladder if you have had an episiotomy. Keep well hydrated so your urine is diluted.
- After going to the toilet pour a jug of warm water over your perineum to rinse it rather than wiping with toilet tissue, then gently dab the area to dry it.
- If you feel constipated and a high-fibre diet and staying hydrated has not helped, ask your midwife or GP about suitable, gentle laxatives.
- The moment you feel the urge to open your bowels, take action right away and sit on the toilet. You can use the second stage breathing – no hard pushing required here either!
- It sounds obvious but do remember to wipe front to back, away from your vagina, to make sure your stitches remain clean.
- Wherever needed, place an ice-pack or ice-cubes, wrapped in a cloth, to relieve discomfort.
- Expose the stitches to fresh air daily to help with the healing process. You can do this by lying on your bed on a towel for 5–10 minutes a couple of times a day.
- Restart your pelvic floor exercises as soon as you can after birth. They enhance blood circulation, and aid the healing process.
- Ask for a referral to a specialist women's health physiotherapist if you feel you would benefit from this. If possible, put some money aside now for a private appointment with an experienced women's health physiotherapist at the six-week mark, as sometimes the NHS waiting

list is quite long. It's very important to take care of your pelvic floor for life – you don't have to accept that when you cough, sneeze or jump you lose a bit of urine. When correctly done, regular pelvic floor exercises will help with any urinary incontinence.

- When you feel ready you could attend a postnatal Pilates class with a well-qualified instructor to help with your core strength. Often there are daytime classes that you can bring your baby along to.

Chapter seventeen

Perineal massage

The perineum is the area between the anus (back passage) and the bottom edge of the vulva. During labour it gets stretched and becomes very thin. This is usual and helps bring about a powerful surge of oxytocin to aid your baby's birth.

Most women tear during labour, but these are usually small and easily repaired, often healing quickly and very well.

The woman's body is perfectly designed to stretch and birth a baby and doesn't require 'preparation'. However, some women find that carrying out perineal massage antenatally gives them confidence. Perineal massage may reduce the likelihood of needing an episiotomy (a cut to the perineum) and may reduce the risk of tearing.

Dr Rachel Reed has written about perineal massage and has an excellent podcast on this topic which I strongly recommend having a listen to.

How to carry out perineal massage

- Start from around 36 weeks.
- Get comfortable, lying against some pillows on the bed, with your legs bent at the knees so you can reach your perineum. You can also try lying on your side and reaching the perineum from underneath your bottom.
- Some women prefer to try perineal massage after they have had a bath and are feeling relaxed.
- Massage a lubricant such as a vegetable-based oil or any plain and unscented carrier oil into the skin of the perineum. There is no need to buy a special perineal massage oil for this purpose, unless you want to.
- Then place your clean thumb (with a short nail) around 3–4cm (or roughly up to the thumb's first knuckle) inside your vagina and press downwards towards the anus.
- Move to each side in a U-shaped stretching movement. This may give a tingling/slightly burning sensation.
- Hold the stretch for 30–60 seconds then release.
- Some find it hard to reach the perineum, in which case your partner can do the massage for you.
- Do not do perineal massage if you have vaginal herpes, thrush or any other vaginal infection.

While perineal massage might not be the most comfortable of things to do, it should not be painful, so if you feel pain stop and try again another time. If you continue to feel pain discuss this with your midwife.

End-of-session summary

- You have now read about all of the different pain management options. With your birth partner or a friend to bounce your thoughts off, why not do a little more research on this, starting with taking a look at the OAA website, which has a pain-relief comparison table and may offer a useful, quick recap of this chapter: www.labourpains. com/assets/_managed/cms/files/InfoforMothers/Pain%20Relief%20 Comparison%20Card/pain%20relief%20comparison%20card%20 september%202014.pdf
- Baby Centre is an excellent and well-referenced resource: www. babycentre.co.uk
- Remember that nothing is set in stone and you can always change your mind on the day.
- We've also covered monitoring and assisted birth and perineal massage. Have a listen to Dr Rachel Reed's podcast on protecting the perineum which is very reassuring: www.birthful.com/podcast-protecting-perineum-tear

"

Let's talk about induction and caesarean birth

"

In the seventh session we talk about:

- What happens when perhaps your due date comes.... and goes. You may be offered an induction of labour, so what is involved, what is the process, what are the pros and cons and are there any natural ways to get things started?

- We'll also look at what happens if you need or wish to request a caesarean birth, and what your recovery may be like.

Chapter eighteen

Due dates and induction of labour

→ It is easy and understandable to become fixated on the estimated due date (EDD) of 40 weeks you have been given to predict your baby's arrival. However, there is no such thing as an exact due date: it is an estimate, which may or may not be accurate, with only around 4-5 percent of babies arriving on their EDD.

Some women gestate their babies for longer than others – and we all develop at different timescales when outside of the womb too. For example, some babies learn to crawl early and others bypass the crawling stage altogether and go straight to walking! And do all apples ripen on a tree on the exact same date, or do some take longer or less time than others?

There are other factors to consider too, such as the length of a woman's menstrual cycle – if your menstrual cycle is longer than the average 28 days your pregnancy may last a little longer too, and vice versa. We are all wonderfully different in many ways and this is the same when it comes to our due dates.

Consider your due date as an estimate rather than something that is set in stone – you may like to think of your baby being due in the first or second half of a particular month, for example.

How are due dates worked out?

Initially your midwife will ask you the date of the first day of your last period. For women with an average length cycle (28 days) that date is considered to be about two weeks before conception. She will then add on 40 weeks from the first day of your last period to generate a due date. Then, at the 12-week ultrasound scan, measurements of the baby are taken and the due date may slightly change to take these into account.

Most babies are born between 37 and 42 weeks of pregnancy (often called 'at term'). So even if you are sure of your conception date, birth can vary by around four weeks.

After 42 weeks there is a small but statistically significant increase in the chance of stillbirth. Even though the rate increases, two Cochrane reviews '...*acknowledge that the risk of stillbirth appears to be very low in longer pregnancies and the latest one suggests it would be necessary to induce 426 women at around 41 to 42 weeks to avoid one stillbirth*' (AIMS – 'Labour induction at term: How great is the risk of refusing it'). For more statistics and in-depth information on this please have a read of the above article and the web links included at the end of this section.

Towards the end of your pregnancy your midwife should offer you information on the risks of stillbirth and also discuss what your options are should you choose to decline induction of labour. There may be other important factors to consider, such as maternal age and health of the mother and baby.

Since there is a small increase in risk past 42 weeks, induction of labour, which is starting labour off using drugs, is usually offered between 41+0 and 42+0 weeks. This varies between hospital Trusts and may differ depending on the woman and/or baby's specific situation. Women are often put under pressure to accept induction, but, like everything, induction isn't risk-free for mother or baby. There are not currently any tests able to predict which babies would be better off inside or induced.

I often hear the words 'They won't let me go past X weeks and are going to induce me'. But the choice to accept or decline induction of labour is always yours. If a woman declines she will be offered additional checks, such as monitoring every 2–3 days when past 42 weeks and an additional ultrasound scan to monitor the depth of the pool of liquor (waters) around the baby – an indication of how the placenta is functioning. You will be invited into hospital to have your baby's heartbeat listened to electronically. But of course all these checks are only useful in that moment. As ever, it is very important to keep monitoring your baby's movements yourself and to get checked out right away if there is any change.

What starts labour?

It is not known exactly how labour starts, but it's thought that the baby sends chemical messages out to signal they are ready to be born. In the last few days of pregnancy some women feel great, while others feel like they have had enough. It can be helpful to remember all the things you and your baby are doing behind the scenes to prepare for the onset of labour, such as:

- Your baby is putting the last finishing touches to the development of their lungs.
- In the third trimester your baby's brain grows faster than ever.
- Your body is preparing for your baby's birth.
- You are passing valuable antibodies to your baby.

How does induction of labour work?

Induction of labour is when your labour is started artificially, using medical methods. There is a non-medical method called a 'membrane sweep', which is an internal examination that your midwife can do to try to encourage labour to start.

Why might you be offered induction of labour

- Your midwife or obstetrician may feel that factors such as your age, weight or any health issues you have mean it is safer to have your labour induced. If this is the case, you can ask for more specific research and information on this – such as statistics for your specific situation – so you are able to make an informed decision.

- Your waters may have released but labour has not started. If your waters release and labour has not started after 24 hours, this can increase the chance of infection, so induction of labour is offered.

It's always good to ask what the *relative* risk of 'X, Y or Z' is versus the *absolute* risk. For example the relative risk of 'X' may be that the risk doubles, but the absolute risk may be that that risk goes from 1 percent to 2 percent, which paints a far less scary picture.

- Your baby may be considered to be 'overdue' (the most common reason for induction is prolonged pregnancy).

But are they really overdue? A study on the AIMS website mentions women who conceived by IVF, who therefore knew when their egg was fertilised, and who found that the routine ultrasound dating scan consistently put their estimated birth date earlier than it should have been by an average of three days. There is a link to this article in the reference section at the back of the book.

Discuss your specific situation with a senior midwife if you feel you're unsure about the due date you've been given.

- Reduced movements. A baby's movements should not slow down or reduce in number.
- The baby's growth rate may be in question. But NICE does not currently recommend induction of labour if a healthcare professional suspects a baby is larger than expected for gestational age (unless there are other factors in place). Growth scans are not always accurate, and some women are told they have a 'big' baby but the baby is born a perfectly average weight.

There are a few different methods of trying to induce your labour, which are usually offered in the following order.

Membrane sweep, or 'stretch and sweep'

In some hospitals a membrane sweep is offered at 40 weeks for a first-time mother and 41 weeks for subsequent babies, and it can be carried out by a midwife or doctor. Membranes are the sac that encases your baby and the amniotic fluid.

If you consent to this procedure, the midwife or doctor will sweep or circle their finger around and inside your cervix. If the cervix is closed the midwife cannot perform a sweep. Sweeps are usually carried out in the venue where you have your usual midwife appointments and you go home as normal afterwards. A sweep can also be carried out as part of the induction process, when you are in the antenatal ward awaiting the start of labour with induction.

Having a sweep can increase the likelihood of either spontaneous labour within 48 hours or delivery within one week. Sweeps are not recommended if your waters have released and labour has not yet started, as this may increase the chance of infection.

Sweeps can be repeated over several days if you wish. A recent Cochrane review states *'Questions remain as to whether there is an optimal number of membrane sweeps and timings and gestation of these to facilitate induction of labour.'* (This study can be found in the reference section). Some women find a membrane sweep uncomfortable or painful and it can cause cramping and bleeding. The woman may have several days of niggly surges, meaning she isn't able to rest as well in the days before her labour starts.

Sometimes during a sweep the midwife may inadvertently break a woman's waters, which has its own set of risks, increasing the chance of infection and meaning the woman is now 'on a clock'.

As with all interventions offered, it's up to you whether you accept or decline a sweep. You can decline a sweep but then request one at a later date.

The process of induction of labour

This is a package that comprises of three parts: prostaglandins, artificial rupture of membranes (releasing a woman's waters) and intravenous synthetic oxytocin, and with this comes the need for regular internal examinations, to see how the cervix is responding (or not) to the drugs given.

As induction of labour can sometimes involve many hours or even a day or so of waiting around you may like to consider a second birth partner. It won't be easy for you or your birth partner to sleep during this time as you will usually be on a busy, noisy antenatal ward. Is there someone other than your partner who could stay with you for the initial few hours/as long as they are needed? That then means that when the actual induction process has begun and your surges are on their way, your partner can join you with fresh energy, ready and energised enough to be able to support you fully, which would be very useful.

Prostaglandin

Prostaglandin is a hormone that helps to soften the cervix and may help start labour by mimicking the natural prostaglandins that do this in preparation for labour. It is inserted into the woman's vagina, behind the cervix. It looks like a pessary (a small almond-shaped tablet) or it can be a gel or sometimes like a small tampon ('propess'). There are several possible side-effects, including hyperstimulation of the uterus, period pain-type sensations, a headache, an irregular heartbeat and feeling sick/ having a bit of an upset stomach.

Midwives can administer prostaglandins on the antenatal ward. They will monitor your baby's heart before and after the procedure. After it has been inserted you will need to rest for around 30–60 minutes to allow it to start being absorbed, and then you can move about or go for a walk.

With the propess, after careful monitoring, it may be suggested that you go home for 24 hours, or until surges start if that is sooner, but not all hospitals offer this as an option.

The process can be repeated again if it does not work, or a caesarean birth may be offered if your doctor feels this may be safer for you and your baby. You can talk through the reasons for recommending a caesarean birth with your doctor and make sure you fully understand why this is being recommended and agree to it.

Sometimes prostaglandins can cause very fast, strong and intense surges (hyperstimulation), which may cause problems for your baby. This is why induction of labour is performed in hospital. If this happens your midwife or doctor will remove the propess if this is what you have had, and/or give you drugs to stop the induction.

Artificial rupture of membranes (ARM) – also known as 'breaking the waters'

This procedure can be carried out by a midwife or doctor and is part of the induction process. It is also sometimes offered to speed up a 'slow' labour (augmentation).

What is the process of ARM?

Your midwife or doctor will make a small break in the membranes surrounding your baby by using a long, thin hook. Ask what the maximum length of time is that you can have after your waters have been released before they commence the synthetic oxytocin drip, as sometimes ARM alone can set labour off, meaning you could potentially skip the next stage of the induction process and carry on 'as you were'. Is it possible you could go for a walk, be gently active then rest on your own for a bit before moving on to the next step?

Intravenous synthetic oxytocin

Synthetic oxytocin is an artificial version of the hormone oxytocin and it is given after ARM if surges have not become established, with dilation of the cervix. Synthetic oxytocin is given through an intravenous drip, which causes more regular surges to establish (ARM alone also causes surges). As it can sometimes cause over-stimulation of the uterus your baby's heart rate will need to be monitored continuously to check that it is within normal limits. It can be adjusted if a problem occurs.

Synthetic oxytocin has quite a few side-effects, similar to prostaglandins, one of which is that it does not allow for a slow build-up of labour surges and endorphins and is therefore likely to be more intense and challenging than a spontaneous labour, so an epidural is offered at the outset. Some women accept this, while others prefer to see how they go and use breathing, gas and air and/or hypnobirthing techniques.

Induction of labour may increase the chance of a woman having an assisted delivery using forceps or ventouse – perhaps because of the increased use of epidurals. In some cases if the induction process fails (the process can fail, not the mother!) the mother may need to have a caesarean birth.

According to NICE '*Induced labour has an impact on the birth experience of women. It may be less efficient and is usually more painful than spontaneous labour, and epidural analgesia and assisted delivery are more likely to be required... Induction of labour has a large impact on the health of women and their babies and so needs to be clearly clinically justified.*'

Sometimes a woman is offered a balloon induction, where a balloon is inserted into the cervix and the balloon is gently filled with fluid to apply pressure to the cervix. The balloon can be kept in place for 12–24 hours and it then either drops out or is taken out, after which it should be possible for the woman's waters to be released.

You may be offered induction of labour via Dilapan. Dilapan is a drug-free rod which is inserted in the cervix, staying for up to 24 hours to expand and start to soften your cervix, after which your waters can be released.

Before you go in for your induction appointment, make sure you eat well and when you arrive, ask the midwife when is the last time you can eat so you can ensure you have plenty of fuel inside you (currently eating is not recommended once a woman has had an epidural set up).

What if induction doesn't work?

You will have a discussion with your obstetrician. They may suggest another try of the induction process, or a caesarean birth may be offered in some circumstances. Some women discuss with the doctor the possibility of having a caesarean rather than continuing with the induction process.

Questions you can ask prior to accepting induction of labour:

- What is the reason I am being offered induction?
- What are the benefits of induction of labour for my specific situation?
- What are the risks (to me or my baby), and how likely are they?
- What pain relief is available and when can I have it?
- What happens if I decline induction of labour?
- If I am booked in for induction and the labour ward fills up with women going into spontaneous labour, what will happen to my appointment? If it will be shifted back this may give you more of an idea how crucial (or not) a particular date is.

Healthcare professionals offering induction of labour should, according to NICE:

- Allow you time to discuss the information with your partner before coming to a decision.
- Encourage you to look at a variety of sources of information.
- Invite you to ask questions, and encourage you to think about your options.

- Support you in whatever decision you make.

When guidelines are written, they are based on the whole nation rather than your specific situation. You should be given personalised information about the benefits and risks for you and your baby, as well as any alternatives.

If you feel unsure about whether or not you want to accept induction of labour, or you don't feel you are being given personalised information, you can request to go through your notes and health background with a senior midwife, consultant midwife or professional maternity advocate (PMA) and make a more personalised plan. To make contact with any of the above just call your main hospital number and ask to be put through to one of them and perhaps ask for an email address too.

One of these experienced midwives will be able to spend time looking at your notes and history and discuss with you the pros and cons of induction of labour for your particular case. Part of their role is to work with you to try to come up with a personalised plan that you are happy with.

Research, research, research – ask as many questions are you need to so you feel comfortable with whatever decision you make.

'Natural' methods of induction of labour

Of course there's no such thing as a 'natural induction', as even these natural methods are still attempting to encourage the baby out before they have signalled they are ready to be born. However, for reasons personal to some, or if you are wanting to avoid a medical induction, the date of which is looming, you may be interested in this section.

Evidence does not support the following methods for induction of labour:

- herbal supplements
- acupuncture
- homeopathy
- castor oil
- hot baths
- enemas
- sexual intercourse

However, it does seem logical that having sex, and in particular the woman having an orgasm, might help. After all, skin-to-skin contact and the female orgasm raise oxytocin levels, and semen in the man's ejaculate has prostaglandins in it. So perhaps it's worth a try, though it's not recommended if your waters have released.

If you have had a straightforward pregnancy you can try nipple/breast stimulation to attempt to help start off labour. When a baby nurses at the breast this produces a big hit of oxytocin and this is what nipple stimulation is trying to recreate. This process works best if the woman's cervix is already 'ripe'. To stimulate the breasts gently rub or roll your nipples and massage the darker area around your nipple (the areola) using your palm in a circular motion, firmly but gently. Focus on one breast at a time and include rest intervals.

Evidence does support breast stimulation to improve cervical ripening (see Evidence Based Birth's article on this, in the reference section), as a way of encouraging labour to start and, interestingly, reducing the rates of postpartum haemorrhage. It's also important to note that there are some cases of reports of nipple stimulation causing hyperstimulation of the uterus, so check with your midwife before doing this.

We are incredibly fortunate to have highly skilled doctors and midwives available to manage induction of labour and other interventions - and they can and do save lives. However, some mothers and healthcare professionals feel that medical methods are overused, and that women are not given clear evidence relevant to their own specific situation to mull over beforehand. It is down to you to ask for this to be provided, if wanted.

If you decide to accept induction of labour, remember that it is possible to have a very positive experience. You can still dim the lights, adjust the room, request as much assistance as possible to remain mobile while being monitored (like having the monitoring equipment set up while you're on the birth ball), and use your breathing and visualisations to keep things as relaxed as possible. There is a MP3 included with this book for induction of labour

The website 'Tell me a good birth story' has positive stories of induction of labour and there are some positive induction of labour Facebook pages too.

The 'before birth' birth plan

When your due date comes... and goes... it can sometimes feel frustrating. It can also become irritating when well-meaning friends and family are constantly asking 'Any news yet?'! After a few days of this anxiety can creep in, potentially raising adrenalin levels, which is not the relaxed state you want to be in as you wait for your body and baby to tip into labour.

If you've already told people your due date, consider telling them that you have had another scan and your due date has now shifted to 7–10 days after the due date you told them. This can take the pressure off and the well-meaning but annoying messages of 'Have you had your baby yet?' or 'Any signs?!' won't start arriving until much later. These well-meaning messages can plant seeds of doubt in your mind – exactly what we don't want.

It can be great to create a 'before birth' birth plan. Choose 14 relaxing things to do to keep you occupied so you're not sat at home just waiting for something to happen.

Here's a suggested plan:

Day 1: Go out for a leisurely lunch or dinner with your partner or a friend.

Day 2: If you'd enjoy it, go to an art gallery/local exhibition or book in for a one-day course.

Day 3: Go to the cinema.

Day 4: Book a relaxing pregnancy massage or maternity reflexology session.

Day 5: Prepare some food such as pasta sauces, soups etc for the freezer in readiness for those early days of parenthood.

Day 6: Do a yoga class then go for tea and cake

Day 7: Meet up with friends/family.

Day 8: Plan a long, local walk with someone.

Day 9: Get a haircut or have a facial, pedicure or some other pampering treat.

Day 10: Have a pyjama day, relaxing and watching lots of comedy – laughter produces feel-good hormones.

Day 11: Declutter the house, go through old photos, do all those odd jobs that will keep you occupied and you won't have time for when the baby arrives.

Day 12: Watch some lovely birth videos and read positive birth stories. If you're so inclined, create a positive birth board for labour.

Day 13: Go for a swim or to an aquanatal class.

Day 14: Take a gentle walk, read a book with your feet up and get a takeaway to have with your partner and have an early night (and perhaps some breast stimulation or other action!).

Chapter nineteen

Caesarean birth

$\rightarrow$ A caesarean birth (also known as caesarean section or c-section) is an operation where the baby is born via an incision in the lower abdomen and uterus. Caesareans can be either planned or unplanned (taking place during labour).

Planned caesareans are usually carried out after 39 weeks unless there is a medical reason to do it sooner. Your date may change if another woman requires a caesarean and her needs are more pressing than yours. If appropriate, you may be able to negotiate waiting until you go into labour.

Most women recover well after a caesarean birth, though there are risks associated with all surgery, and it will take longer to get 'back to normal' afterwards.

Currently, in the UK, caesarean birth is not recommended unless there is a medical reason that makes it necessary. If a woman is being refused a caesarean for non-medical reasons, guidance states that she should be referred on to another obstetrician or hospital more open to carrying out a maternal request caesarean.

For some women it is recommended that they give birth via caesarean. Reasons could include:

- Placental issues such as placenta praevia (when the placenta covers the outlet) or placental abruption (when the placenta starts to come away from the uterus wall).
- Medical issues such as raised blood pressure (pre-eclampsia).
- Your baby's position – if your baby is lying transverse or oblique (horizontally) or is breech (although some women choose to opt for a vaginal breech birth).
- If your baby is in a breech position doctors may offer to try to turn your baby into a head-down position using pressure on your abdomen. This procedure is called an ECV (external cephalic version) and is usually offered at around 36 weeks of pregnancy. It has about a 50 percent success rate. Some babies just turn back, as perhaps this is the right position for them!
- Multiple pregnancy – although some women have vaginal twin or triplet births.
- If labour is not progressing and the woman agrees to a caesarean for this.
- Severe growth restriction.

If your baby is in a breech position ask your midwife about moxibustion – a type of Chinese acupuncture which may be effective from 34–36 weeks of pregnancy. Moxa are little sticks of dried herbs which are lit, then the flame is blown out leaving the stick smoking and hot. It is then placed near the little toe, at the base, to heat very specific energy points there. Then you switch to the other foot. Heat is absorbed into the energy points via energy channels, triggering hormonal changes which relax the muscles of the uterus. This means there is a little more space in the uterus, which in turn will increase your baby's activity, hopefully encouraging them to turn. According to Denise Tiran, moxibustion has around a 66 percent success rate, so it may be worth a shot if your baby is breech and you're hoping they will turn head down. Some hospitals offer moxibustion, or you can arrange it privately with an acupuncturist. Always check with your midwife or doctor before attempting moxibustion as it's not always appropriate, for example if you have a low-lying placenta, high blood pressure or excess amniotic fluid.

Or perhaps you have no desire to try to encourage your baby to turn and instead are happy to opt for a planned caesarean or a vaginal breech birth.

Some women are anxious about giving birth vaginally, for a variety of reasons, including having a fear of childbirth (tokophobia). Others are worried their partner may miss the birth as he or she will be away when they are due.

If you have a lot of anxiety or fear around giving birth you can discuss this with your midwife who may offer to refer you to a perinatal mental health specialist to talk it through. If a woman continues to ask for a caesarean birth her wishes should be respected.

What are the risks for caesarean birth?

All surgery carries risks and we all view risk differently. Risk is very personal and our feelings about it can be dependent on past experiences and how we personally view things.

If a woman is healthy and well the risks are reduced. The main risks of giving birth by caesarean are:

- Wound infection – this is common. It can take some time for the wound to heal, perhaps several weeks.
- Blood clots developing in the legs – which may travel up into the lungs. To help try to prevent this compression stockings are usually issued and sometimes blood-thinning injections which the mother self-administers for a few days after birth.
- Heavy bleeding.
- Damage to internal organs such as the bladder or bowel.
- Babies born by caesarean may need assistance with breathing or require time in the special care baby unit.
- Babies are at a small risk of being cut during the procedure (1–2 in 100), though this is usually not deep and heals well.
- Any risks that the anaesthetic used may bring.

A first caesarean is usually a relatively simple operation, but subsequent caesareans are not so predictable, due to the scar tissue that remains from the previous surgery. If a woman has had a caesarean for her first baby (or subsequent babies) she can choose to have a vaginal birth next time if she wishes and this is called a VBAC (vaginal birth after caesarean).

What happens during a caesarean?

The exact procedure can vary from hospital to hospital.

- The woman needs to read and sign a consent form before the operation.
- She will need to put on a hospital gown, remove any jewellery and contact lenses and sometimes she is asked to remove nail polish (so the nail bed can be viewed easily to check oxygen blood levels).
- If the caesarean is not an emergency she usually receives a regional anaesthetic, which can be given via an epidural if one is already in place, or by spinal, which is similar to an epidural but quicker acting. The drugs given mean she will not feel any pain, but she will feel some sensation, like a tugging, which is normal.
- She will be awake and clear headed for her baby's birth.
- Sometimes a woman has the procedure under a general anaesthetic and in these cases partners cannot come into the theatre.

There are lots of people present at a caesarean birth, usually at least eight or more, so don't be alarmed when you see the room fill up as this is normal.

As a rough guide, your baby will be born within around 10-15 minutes and the rest of the operation takes around 45 minutes to an hour, longer for multiple births or for when things are less straightforward.

The placenta is removed during the procedure. It is usually possible to have optimal cord clamping, though it won't be for the full 10-20 minutes. Do mention this in advance so the team are aware.

You can hold your baby right away providing they do not require any immediate medical attention. Some mothers choose to breastfeed while in theatre, while others prefer to wait until they are in the recovery room.

Lots and lots of skin-to-skin with the baby after birth is always good and will also help your milk 'come in' if you're planning on breastfeeding. Ask your midwife for help with holding positions that won't touch or knock your lower abdomen.

Parent/baby-centred/natural approach to caesarean birth

If of interest, you can ask about a natural approach caesarean, sometimes called a 'mother-centred' or 'baby-centred' caesarean. The following points may or may not be an option and it is something it would ideally be best to talk through in advance, if at all possible.

During a parent/baby caesarean your own music or a hypnobirthing MP3 can be played during the operation. The drape is removed or lowered and the head of the bed is raised so you can see your baby being born, rather than the doctor doing this speedily. Once the incision has been made, as the baby's head becomes visible the surgeon is hands off. The baby breathes air for the first time while their trunk is still in the uterus, attached to the placental blood flow. This delay of a few minutes helps the baby to release lung liquid, which is what happens during a vaginal birth. The baby's shoulders are then eased out. As the baby emerges, you can discover the sex yourself. They are then placed on you for immediate skin-to-skin.

What is recovery like after a caesarean?

After an hour or so in the recovery area, where the mother, her partner and her baby go, assuming the baby doesn't require any medical assistance, the mother is transferred to a postnatal ward where she will stay for 1–3 days, depending on her specific situation. She often feels uncomfortable for the first 2–3 days and painkillers are offered. It gets easier over time with full recovery time varying from woman to woman. Keep on top of the timings of your aftercare medication so the relief is consistent.

Keeping mobile helps with managing any pain or discomfort. Try to stand up straight and gently change your position from time to time.

The wound can feel sore for a few weeks after the operation.

Some women suffer with trapped wind pain or difficulty urinating – talk to your midwife if this happens. There is some evidence that chewing gum within 24 hours after birth may help with bowel recovery. Some women find peppermint tea soothing to drink.

Take a few deep breaths every hour to clear your lungs and when coughing, sneezing or laughing, bend your legs or hold a pillow over your tummy to help with discomfort.

You should be given some information on gentle exercises to do – ask for this if you don't get it.

As with after any birth it is important to take it easy and not be in a rush to get back to normal. If you had your appendix out, or any other operation, would you rush back to work and back to normal? We tend to expect mothers to get back to normal (whatever 'normal' is!) quickly after birth, including a caesarean birth, which puts too much pressure on them at a time when they should ideally be resting as much as possible.

Avoid strenuous exercise and driving for around six weeks (just like you would after any operation). Check with your GP and car insurance if you want to drive sooner than this. You can always ask about these things at your six-week GP check, which is an appointment to see how you and your baby are doing. Remember the scar will heal from the outside in, so even when the scar looks like it's well healed, there will still be a lot of healing going on behind the scenes.

If you had an unplanned caesarean you may feel mixed emotions and question why things did not go as you had hoped they would. You can arrange to talk through your birth with a midwife to get answers and explanations, which may help you feel at peace with what happened and why. This service is available for all women, regardless of what type of birth they had – you just need to request it.

In the UK it's fairly standard for partners to get two weeks' leave from work after their baby's birth. Who can you call upon after this time to help you with things, or who can pop by to support and nurture you and maybe bring food and take over a bit so you can rest? Is a postnatal doula a suggestion that could work for you if needed?

In the event of a planned caesarean birth

- Prepare lots of questions in advance and ideally speak with the anaesthetist as well as the surgeon. Will the people you are talking to be the same ones carrying out your caesarean, and if not, how will they ensure your wishes are heard by the relevant staff?
- Request that if possible you have one of the early morning appointments as there is less likelihood of waiting around then, or for delays.

- If you would like to walk into the theatre rather than be wheeled in (this can apply for an unplanned caesarean too if wanted), discuss this with staff.
- You can still use your hypnobirthing techniques and MP3s – they will be invaluable in keeping you calm as you wait around before you are prepped to go to theatre, as well as during your baby's birth.

Please see the next chapter for a caesarean birth plan template.

End-of-session summary

- We've now looked at due dates and induction of labour and why you may be offered it. We've also considered what might be involved in a caesarean birth. I'd like to invite you to read more deeply into these topics, and perhaps make notes about what your preferences would be in these situations.
- Here is the article on the evidence for induction of labour: evidencebasedbirth.com/evidence-on-due-dates
- There is also a lot of information to be found here: www.sarawickham.com/topic-resources/post-term-pregnancy-and-induction-of-labour-resources
- This article may be useful for preparing for a caesarean and knowing what to expect: www.labourpains.com/assets/_managed/cms/files/InfoforMothers/C-SECTION/Labour-Pains-Caesarean-Section-Information-sheet-EN.pdf
- You may like to do a little research on Vitamin K as this gets offered to your baby soon after birth: www.sarawickham.com/topic-resources/a-decade-of-vitamin-k-articles and evidencebasedbirth.com/evidence-for-the-vitamin-k-shot-in-newborns
- We discuss the process of making birth plans in the next session. Remember that however your birth unfolds, your preferences are important and should be taken seriously by your caregivers.

"

Let's talk about feeding your baby, making a birth plan and postnatal recovery

"

In the eighth session we talk about:

- Feeding your baby. We'll discuss how breastfeeding works and how you can get things off to a good start if you choose to breastfeed, and look at how you can access support if things aren't going well. We also look at what you'll need if you choose to breastfeed or formula feed.

- Some decisions about infant feeding may need to be included on your birth plan, so next we'll look at how to put plans A, B and C in place so that you are prepared for whatever happens at your birth.

- Finally, we'll consider healing and rest after birth. How can you prepare now for this and who can you call upon to help once your baby is here? How will you handle visitors? There's a general overview of your physical recovery and what to look out for, and discussion of your and your partner's all-important mental health.

Chapter twenty

Feeding your baby

→ This chapter* touches on information about feeding your baby, helps you make decisions, guides you as you initiate feeding and signposts you to support and further information should you want it. Recommended further reading is included at the end of the book, along with websites to expand on the information included here.

How breastfeeding works

Babies are born with the innate ability to breastfeed and, with rare exceptions, mothers are excellent at making milk. Feeding your baby requires responsiveness and believing in your ability to do it!

Your baby's feeds in the first few days are hormone driven: the first milk, colostrum, is made during pregnancy and is ready to feed your baby immediately following birth. After two to five days, mature milk 'comes in',

---

* This chapter was contributed by breastfeeding counsellor Kate Cameron: www.katecameronbreastfeeding.co.uk

thanks to delivery of your placenta causing changes in your hormones and your baby suckling to stimulate the milk supply. Then lactation becomes driven by your baby: your breasts make milk according to your baby's needs, hence the 'supply and demand' effect. The more you feed your baby/express your milk, the more milk you make.

Breastmilk gives your baby all the nutrition and hydration (and more!) that they need for approximately the first six months of life. (Breastmilk is approximately 87 percent water.)

Skin-to-skin contact as much as possible following birth and in the early weeks is beneficial for milk supply stimulation, effective attachment and milk transfer. As you cuddle your baby, you both benefit from oxytocin release, encouraging feelings of bonding and promoting lactation.

It takes approximately six to eight weeks to establish breastfeeding, by which time your breasts will have learned to respond to your baby's needs, settling down to making the right amount of milk for them, and your baby will have learned to feed effectively. In the meantime, following your baby's cues and feeding them whenever they show interest and for however long they want to feed, will satisfy your baby's needs and encourage your breasts to match them.

Preparing to breastfeed

When planning to breastfeed your baby, you may consider purchasing a few items:

- A few crop-top-style or comfortable traditional-style nursing bras, without underwires or padding
- Muslins
- Breast pads
- Nipple cream
- Breast pump (see Expressing section below)
- A breastfeeding pillow

Being fitted for a nursing bra at around 37 weeks of pregnancy means a reasonable estimate of your final size can be made. You could make a fitting appointment with a department store or bra specialist. Nursing crop-tops can be comfortable and supportive for breastfeeding in the initial few weeks, especially when you spend a lot of time at home.

They are also more generally sized than bras so exact measuring is not necessary. A few weeks after your baby is born, you could arrange an accurate fitting when you are ready to purchase more bras.

Muslins are useful when burping, to catch any posseting (which is when a baby brings up a little milk) and mop up leaky breasts or baby's leaky mouth! You will need lots of these, so a pack of four will not cut it.

It is normal for your breasts to leak, particularly in the first few weeks before breastfeeding is established. You may need to change your breast pads frequently during this time. Breast pads can be disposable or reusable. If using washable breast pads, you will need at least six pairs.

Nipples are a sensitive part of your body, and in the first few days following your baby's birth they can feel particularly sensitive. This is partly thanks to the serum secreted from the glands (known as 'Montgomery tubercles') on your areolae, surrounding your nipples. This serum cleanses and lubricates your nipples, preparing them for breastfeeding. Your baby's suckling may cause your nipples to feel sensitive, but if your nipple is not being misshapen, pinched or damaged during feeding, this sensitivity is normal and will ease after the first week or so. Lanolin-based creams or vegan alternatives applied after feeding can be soothing and promote healing. They do not usually need to be washed off before the next feed, but check the instructions on the packaging.

A breastfeeding cushion may be helpful for some feeding positions or after a caesarean birth, to support your baby's weight and take the pressure off your abdomen, scar area or back and arms. You might want to read reviews to help you choose one.

Initiating breastfeeding

Within the first hour of being born, babies are at their most alert, giving the perfect opportunity for offering the first feed. If there are any interruptions to the process of being born, placed skin-to-skin with mum and suckling, your baby can be offered skin-to-skin and a feed as soon as you are both ready.

Babies can crawl and wriggle their way to the breasts when placed on their mother's abdomen or chest and are attracted by the smell of the serum secreted from around the nipples, the smell of colostrum, the sound of their mother's heartbeat and the sight of the usually darker nipple against the paler skin of the breast. Like all mammals, babies are born with the ability to suckle (from approximately 34 weeks gestation) and they will use their head bobbing reflex to self-attach, often trying several times before they get it right! This is known as latching on. Sometimes babies require a little guidance to latch on, but it is worth being patient and letting them figure it out by themselves if they can. Over-handling of a newly born baby's head, which may be feeling sore and bruised, should be avoided.

After the first feed, babies need time to recover from labour and birth, giving parents a chance to rest too. During the first 24 hours following birth, your baby will enjoy and benefit from skin-to-skin time with both parents, with frequent access to the breasts to enable baby to latch on should they want to. Your baby's tummy capacity will be small in the first 24 hours, approximately 5ml, the equivalent of a teaspoon.

After those first 24 hours, your baby will feed more frequently as they start to recover from the birth and feel more wakeful, still enjoying the emotional and physical benefits of skin-to-skin contact. Up to approximately six weeks old, feeding may take from five to 45 minutes, between eight and 12 times per day (every two to three hours).

When your baby is around two to five days old, your mature milk will start to 'come in'. Your baby's stomach capacity will increase to accommodate the larger volume of milk, to approximately 15ml, equivalent to one tablespoon. This can be an emotional time for mothers (known as the 'baby blues') as hormone levels change and there is a dramatic fall in oestrogen. The breasts may feel heavy, hard and painful too. This is known as engorgement and is due to increased blood supply to the breasts, to transport the nutrients for milk-making, increased lymph fluid and your glandular tissue swelling as your milk is produced faster than your baby can use it. There are some self-help measures which may relieve you:

- Gentle breast massage: try using circular motion all round your breasts or combing your knuckles towards your nipples.
- A warm compress before feeding to help the milk flow.
- A cold compress/ice pack to relieve the swelling.
- Paracetamol or ibuprofen (both are suitable for breastfeeding mothers).
- Place chilled cabbage leaves against your breasts for their anti-inflammatory effect.

- Offer your baby your breast frequently.
- Express a small amount of milk by hand to soften the area around your nipple, making it easier for your baby to latch on. Resist the temptation to express any more than this as it will encourage your breasts to replenish to the same level: the more you express, the more you encourage milk production.

Engorgement should ease after a few days and your breasts will become more comfortable. You will notice lumpy pockets of milk filling up between feeds, and your breasts will feel softened and smoother after feeds. Initially babies tend to feed from one breast at each feed, so you alternate the breast you offer. If your baby sometimes or always wants to feed from both breasts, you alternate the breast you start on at each feed, to roughly balance stimulation on both sides. From a few weeks old babies may feed from both breasts at some or all feeds.

Allowing your baby to feed as often and for as long as they want will encourage your milk supply to match their needs. This is known as responsive feeding. Feeding cues include head bobbing and trying to latch on when being held, lip and mouth movements, lip smacking, poking the tongue out, hand to mouth movements and fist or finger suckling.

Non-nutritive suckling is soothing for babies, enabling them to release oxytocin to help relieve pain and make them feel loved and secure.

Positioning and attachment

There are many ways to hold your baby at the breast and you may vary the position you use from feed to feed, or you may choose one position that works well for you. Your feeding position needs to be comfortable so that you can maintain it for as long as your baby takes to feed. Some mothers use cushions and pillows for support, a lower back cushion, a foot stool or piece of furniture to rest their feet on, or they raise their lap by simply bending their knees when feeding in bed or outstretched on the sofa. After a caesarean birth it can be more challenging to get comfortable when feeding: some mothers like to use pillows to support their baby's weight across their body, while others prefer the underarm (or rugby) hold where the baby rests on a cushion, tucked into his mother's side, away from her abdomen and scar area. Side-lying can be restful, and is particularly useful following a caesarean birth or vaginal stitches.

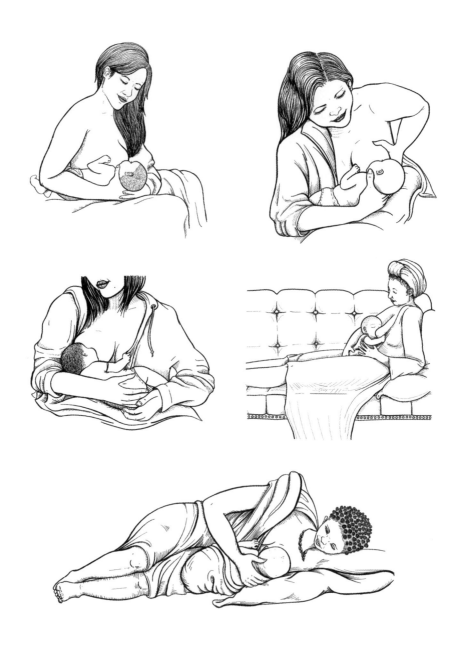

Your baby can feed in any position that is comfortable and allows them to reach the breast easily. They should be snuggled close against your body with their chin in line with their breastbone and their head tilted back slightly. Your baby's head should be free to move, rather than held rigidly by your hand.

If you need to, you can support your baby by placing the heel of your hand against their shoulder blades with your finger and thumb gently touching the bony part behind his ears.

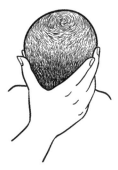

When your baby starts to open their mouth widely as they approach the breast, their chin and lower lip should come into contact with your breast first, with their lower lip curled outwards as their chin indents the breast. Their top lip then reaches over the nipple and attaches to the breast closer to the nipple than the bottom lip. This is an off-centre latch, where the nipple is encouraged towards the roof and the back of your baby's mouth.

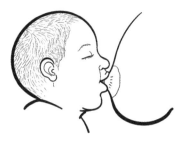

shallow latch (incorrect)

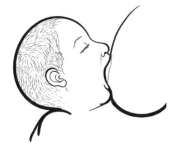

deep latch (correct)

A comfortable off-centre latch will encourage efficient milk transfer and you may hear your baby swallowing. A latch that remains painful after the first 30 seconds or so probably needs adjusting. You can take your baby off the breast by gently inserting your little finger (with a short nail!) into the corner of your baby's mouth to break the suction.

Sometimes it can be challenging for a little newborn to latch on to a full breast, so you can make it easier by shaping the breast using your hand in a C or U-shape (depending on the angle of your baby's approach to the breast). Flattening the breast between your thumb and fingers and tilting it so that the nipple is angled towards the roof of your baby's mouth can help them latch more deeply. Your thumb will be close to your nipple, indenting your breast and causing your nipple to angle towards your thumb. When you are flattening your breast (imagine flattening a thick sandwich or hamburger to get your mouth into it!), your hand needs to be in the right position – pointing the nipple into the roof of your baby's mouth, not into the side of his cheek. Generally, this means using a U-shape for the cradle, cross cradle and under arm ('rugby ball') holds, and a C-shape for laid-back breastfeeding, side-lying and when baby is vertically sitting on your lap, leaning against your abdomen, breast and perhaps your upper arm too.

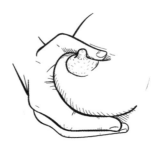

Signs that breastfeeding is going well

Babies who are doing well with breastfeeding will show several daily signs to indicate that they are thriving and stimulating your breasts to make the right amount of milk for them. These are:

- Feeding at least eight times in 24 hours, after the first two days
- Settling contentedly after feeds
- 6–8 wet nappies per 24 hours, from one week old
- 2–3 soiled nappies per day from one week old. (As long as they are not in pain, it is normal for breastfed babies from one week old to go for up to 10 days without a bowel movement.)
- Soft yellow stools from one week old
- Breasts feel fuller before a feed and softer afterwards

The first stools are black meconium, followed by a greenish brown stool caused by colostrum being digested. By one week old babies should produce yellow liquid stools.

Feeds may last from five to 45 minutes in the first few weeks, usually getting shorter as babies practise suckling and become more efficient at transferring milk. The length of feeds will also vary depending on whether your baby is just thirsty or ready for a hunger-satisfying meal. Incidentally, breastfed babies do not need to be given water to drink, even in hot weather. In hot weather formula-fed babies may need water to drink, which should be cooled boiled tap water for babies under six months old.

A baby's weight gain can be a helpful indicator of successful feeding over a period of time. However, babies may adjust to their genetic size during the first few months of life, causing them to keep us on our toes as they move up or down the percentile curves. Be mindful not to get too hung up on growth charts, but to watch for daily signs that your baby is thriving. It is normal and expected for babies to drop up to 10 percent of their birth weight in the first few days of life, usually regaining it by between 10 days and three weeks.

Coping with common problems

Initial problems with feeding may include:

- Sore nipples
- Perceived low milk supply
- Frequent feeding
- Cluster feeding
- Too much milk
- Breast engorgement
- Blocked ducts
- Mastitis
- Thrush
- Tongue-tie

As discussed above, sore nipples are usually a sign of your baby's latch needing improving or adjusting. It is recommended that you seek support from a breastfeeding specialist who can observe you feeding and make suggestions for improving your comfort. Seeking support is discussed later in this chapter.

Some mothers worry about their milk supply, especially if their baby wants to feed frequently or they feel as though their breasts are sometimes empty. Mothers are designed to feed more than one baby and almost all women can make enough milk for their baby (and twins or multiples). If a mother has low levels of prolactin or glandular tissue, she may not be able to produce all of the milk her baby needs. These are rare conditions. Previous breast surgery could also affect breastfeeding.

Sometimes a difficult birth, perhaps requiring medical intervention, a challenging time in the first few days, stress, tiredness or feeling unwell, can impact on the beginning of your breastfeeding journey. However, establishing breastfeeding can take several weeks, so there is enough time to overcome problems.

It is normal for breasts to feel fuller and less full at different times of the day, often in conjunction with your levels of prolactin, which vary throughout the day and night. The breasts are constantly replenishing your milk supply as your baby feeds and between feeds, so the more your baby feeds, the more of your milk they will transfer. Staying well hydrated, eating to hunger and resting as you need to will help to ensure you look after yourself, and your breasts look after your baby's needs.

Sometimes babies want to feed frequently, and it is easier to cope if you understand why and are expecting it! Their tummies are tiny, breastmilk is absorbed easily, babies go through growth spurts/hungry days and their little bodies need frequent hydration and nourishment. To be prepared for frequent feeding frenzies you might want to have a feeding area set up with everything you need within arm's reach, such as your bottle of water, snacks, pillows, foot stool, muslins, breast pads, nipple cream, nappy changing equipment, remote control, mobile phone, glass of wine (yes, you can!) and so on.

Cluster feeding can sound demanding: parents imagine hours of constant feeding with a baby never giving his wilting mother a break! Cluster feeding is normal in the early weeks and months, usually in the evenings, but can take place at any time of day. The feeds are typically close together, with your baby alternating between breasts several times. Your baby may be filling up for a long stretch of sleep ahead (hopefully) or making up for the typically lower levels of prolactin in the evening, which may make your milk flow more slowly. During this time a baby can be fussy at the breast and unsettled, even though they are happy during the rest of the day and not in pain. It might feel tempting to supplement with a bottle of formula during cluster feeding sessions, but beware that supplementing is likely to give your breasts the message to make less milk.

Too much milk can be inconvenient and uncomfortable for a mother and make feeding stressful and overwhelming for the baby, as they cough and splutter their way through a forceful feed. If you have too much milk, you could try to resist the temptation to express, as this will encourage more milk! However, expressing a small amount before feeding your baby may take away the forcefulness of your let down, enabling them to start feeding without choking on the milk. Also, upright feeding positions where your baby leans vertically against you can make a fast flow more manageable for your baby.

Block feeding is a technique sometimes used to help reduce an over-abundant milk supply: only one breast is offered during a three-hour period, regardless of how many times the baby wants to feed. For the following three hours, or block, the other breast is offered. Block feeding for up to a week can help to reduce milk supply by reducing the stimulation to each breast in turn.

We've already discussed breast engorgement under initiating breastfeeding, but engorgement can also happen later in your breastfeeding journey, perhaps if a feed or expressing session is missed, or if weaning off the breast happens too rapidly. Weaning is discussed further on in this chapter.

Breastmilk is made in the glandular tissue, then travels through the milk ducts to the nipple. There are between four and 18 ductal openings in the nipple. If a milk duct becomes blocked, milk may back up behind the blockage, causing a painful lump. Blocked ducts can be relieved with self-help measures such as a warm compress and massage, followed by feeding your baby with their chin on or as close as possible to the blocked area. Alternating breasts, frequent feeding and wearing a gently supportive and well-fitted bra can help to reduce the risk of blocked ducts. Keeping in touch with your breasts both before and after feeds can help to identify problems early. Breasts feel lumpy with pockets of milk before a feed and smoother after a feed. A blocked duct will continue to feel like a hard lump after a feed.

Mastitis is inflammation of the breast tissue, often occurring as a result of a blocked duct not being treated. It may show as a red rash on the affected area and feel hot and particularly tender. Non-infected mastitis can be treated in the same way as a blocked duct. Mothers with infected mastitis usually feel unwell with a fever and flu-like symptoms and need to take a course of antibiotics. Pain relief such as paracetamol and ibuprofen can be taken to reduce temperature and inflammation. It is important to continue feeding from the affected side to help clear the blockage and prevent more from forming.

Thrush on your nipples and in your baby's mouth can be treated with anti-fungal cream and oral drops. Signs of thrush include shiny, painful or itchy nipples, both during and after feeding, white patches in your baby's mouth, nappy rash and fussing at the breast as their mouth feels sore. Taking precautions to help prevent thrush includes good hand hygiene, changing breast pads regularly and ensuring your baby is attached well so that your nipples do not become cracked.

Tongue-tie (Ankyloglossia)

The frenulum is the membrane that attaches the tongue to the floor of the mouth. A short or tight frenulum or one that is attached too close to the tip of the tongue can affect a baby's ability to maintain the latch, suckle effectively, or at all. Sometimes tongue-tie causes pain for the mother. In some cases, the restricted mobility barely affects feeding and the tongue-tie stretches naturally with breastfeeding experience. For other babies, tongue-tie division may be necessary. The website of the Association of Tongue Tie Practitioners lists the qualified practitioners in your area.

Night feeding

Having your baby sleeping close by will minimise disturbance for you all: quiet response when they stir, low lighting if any, minimal talking and avoiding a nappy change or two if it's not necessary, and if you can feed while lying down, is all the better for you! Being woken for feeds at night can be tiring, so catching up during the day with power naps when your baby is sleeping will help you cope with broken sleep.

Expressing and storing breastmilk

If breastfeeding cannot start immediately for any reason, such as mother and baby being temporarily separated for special care, colostrum can be expressed by hand into a 1ml syringe. Your baby can be finger-fed with the syringe alongside your middle finger, gently squeezing the colostrum into their mouth as they suckle, to help them prepare for breastfeeding. Once your mature milk comes in, your baby may be ready to feed at the breast. If not, you can continue to express, perhaps moving on to using a pump, and feed your baby via the finger-feeding tube technique (a nasogastric tube inserted into your baby's mouth alongside your middle finger) to encourage a strong and deep suckling action, imitating as far as possible that used for breastfeeding. It can be helpful to avoid bottle teats in the early weeks to prevent nipple-teat confusion. Once feeding is established (usually around 6-8 weeks), some parents decide to give their babies a bottle of expressed milk, occasionally or regularly. Expressing from this time means that your milk supply will not be over-stimulated by the addition of an expressing session and your baby is more likely to adjust smoothly when switching from breast to bottle teat and back again.

Because of varying prolactin levels, it can be easier to express earlier in the day rather than towards the evening. The amount of milk you express is not indicative of how much milk your baby takes when they breastfeed: it can be difficult to create let downs with a plastic pump with which you do not have an emotional relationship, and mothers with excellent milk supply for their babies may find expressing a challenge.

Breastmilk can be stored at room temperature for up to six hours, in the fridge at four degrees C or cooler for up to one week and in the freezer (in zip-lock milk bags) at -18 degrees C for up to six months.

The various types of pumps available include hands-free silicone suction pumps, manual pumps, single and double electric and hands-free electric. It might seem difficult to choose in advance of your baby's arrival, because you do not know yet when or if you will need or want to express. Colostrum is expressed by hand, so you're covered there. If you need to express your mature milk while still in hospital, you will be provided with a hospital-grade pump, with a ready-sterilised collection kit. If you need to express your milk once you are home with your baby, you may want to buy or hire an electric pump. A double pump can be useful if you need to express every feed for your baby, such as for babies in special care. For occasional expressing to boost your milk supply or give your baby small top-up feeds, a manual pump might be suitable.

Sometimes mothers are recommended to express some colostrum ahead of their baby's arrival (known as harvesting), for example when they have gestational diabetes or are expecting multiples. Antenatal expression of colostrum is done in the same way as it would be after your baby is born if you or he were unable to breastfeed straight away: massaging and gently squeezing a few droplets into a syringe, and storing in the freezer until needed.

Mixed feeding/weaning

Once breastfeeding is established, some parents decide to introduce occasional or regular formula feeds. Regular formula feeds should be introduced gradually, offering one bottle of formula in place of a breastfeed for a few days before introducing a second formula feed. This gives the breasts a chance to adjust gently to reduced stimulation and helps to prevent blocked ducts and mastitis. You could continue increasing the formula feeds and decreasing breastfeeds until the desired balance is reached, or continue until your baby is fully weaned from the breast. You may want to read about your baby's gut microbiome before introducing formula.

Partners

When a baby is feeding frequently and lengthily in the early weeks, their other parent may wonder when he/she gets a look in. How does the non-feeding parent have opportunities to bond with the baby and one-to-one time to get to know each other? Forming a connection with your baby in the early days and weeks is equally vital for both parents and different forms of communication are used in the process: verbal communication (babies love hearing you sing, so you could revise a few nursery rhymes ahead of your baby's arrival if you've forgotten them from your own childhood!), eye contact, facial expression and physical contact. All these methods of communication can be used when their other parent is winding and settling baby after feeds, having skin-to-skin time with baby, changing their nappy or bathing and massaging them. Partners may enjoy 'wearing' baby in a sling around the home or out and about.

Formula feeding

If you decide to formula feed your baby, or breastfeeding does not work out for you, you will need bottles and teats, a sterilising kit and infant formula powder. Formula is available in cartons as a liquid, which is convenient for your hospital bag but more expensive.

Formula companies follow standards and all brands contain the same vital ingredients, so when it comes to choosing, you could opt for the cheapest. Formula is a cows' milk product, altered to be suitable for babies. First stage or infant milk is suitable until your baby is one year old, and there is no benefit to using so-called 'follow-on milk'. When preparing formula feeds it is important to follow the instructions exactly, with regards to safe preparation and quantities. If you have any questions regarding formula preparation, you could have a chat with your midwife or health visitor.

Responsive feeding is important for bottle-fed babies too, regardless of whether there is breast or formula milk in the bottle. Try not to encourage your baby to 'finish' a bottle – watch them carefully and stop when they show signs of having had enough. UNICEF has good information about responsive bottle-feeding on its website.

Seeking support

There are several avenues of support available to parents wanting breastfeeding information, questions answered, emotional support, or practical tips while being observed feeding or just a chat to find out what is normal. There are some excellent evidence-based websites and books on breastfeeding (see resources at the end of the book).

Following your baby's birth, midwives and/or maternity support workers will be on hand and once you are discharged from your community midwifery team, your health visitors can support you with anything baby-related, including feeding. You may want to talk to your GP about breastfeeding, particularly if there are any medical issues.

Before your baby's arrival you may like to research and visit your free-of-charge local drop-in breastfeeding support groups to see which might suit you.

Breastfeeding specialists such as breastfeeding counsellors, lactation consultants (IBCLCs) and peer supporters can give support over the telephone, face to face or via social media.

There are national helplines operating seven days a week. (See their websites for more details.)

- National Breastfeeding helpline 0300 100 0212
- NCT Helpline 0300 330 0700
- The Association of Breastfeeding Mothers 0300 330 5453
- La Leche League 0345 120 2918

For a detailed list of further information about feeding, see the references section at the end of the book.

Chapter twenty-one

Birth plans/birth preferences

→ You don't have to write a birth plan, but many people choose to. You can follow a template such as the NHS one which is available online or create your own. Your midwife may give you one or a template may be in your handheld notes – if your notes are still the handheld version.

It can be helpful to write your birth preferences sheet with your birth partner so he or she is aware of your hopes and wishes. During the active phase of labour when surges are at their most powerful you may not want to talk, so if your partner is aware of what you want it can help you to focus only on yourself.

Some may say 'What's the point of writing a birth plan, it all goes out the window anyway?' – but why would you not plan for and think about what you might like to happen during the biggest, most important thing you will ever do? A big part of writing a birth plan is that it helps you become aware of all of your options and choices.

Yes, birth can be unpredictable, which is why being very flexible and planning for different eventualities can be useful – so you might like to devise a plan A – straightforward birth wishes, B – induction thoughts and C – caesarean wishes. Once you have written your birth plan, put aside any concerns and spend time and effort focusing on the birth you want and not on the 'what ifs'. If the 'what ifs' happen, not only will you have highly skilled midwives with you to help, but you will also have prepared for them and thought about what you would want in that situation, which afterwards can help you feel more at peace with how things went.

Ideas to think about for your birth preferences

If you have practised using hypnobirthing you can put a short section at the front of the birth plan mentioning this. You can then add in some or all of the following, as you see fit. Some of these suggestions might not appeal to you, in which case you can just omit them.

Using bullet points and keeping it to one page for each plan is helpful. Bring along several copies and your birth partner can ensure it gets read. In the unlikely event that you feel your birth preferences are not being taken seriously, ask to change midwife! No one should be making light of your hopes and wishes.

- Where possible, please direct any questions to my birth partner initially so I can stay in my zone.
- If mother and baby are doing well we'd prefer to allow the birth to take its time.
- I would like a dimly-lit, quiet environment and want to give birth at home/on the midwife-led unit/on the labour ward.
- Please don't offer me pain relief. If this is something I would like I will ask for it at the time. OR, my pain relief options are.... in order of preference (list your preferences).
- I would like to be encouraged to keep active and use equipment like a birth ball, birth stool or bean bags.
- In the absence of a medical emergency, please do not offer coached pushing at the second stage. I would like a quiet and calm environment so I can follow my body's lead to birth my baby.
- I would not like student midwives or doctors in with me, OR I am happy to have students (as a side note, many women report having had a fantastic experience with student midwives!)
- I would not like any vaginal examinations (remember you can always

change your mind about this, or anything else) OR, I would like just one initial assessment, OR I am happy to have regular examinations. Perhaps you'd like to ask that your partner gets told how dilated you are so they relay this information to you in their encouraging words. Or maybe you'd simply rather be told whether or not you're progressing well and not know numbers.

- I would like to try the birth pool.
- If I choose to have an epidural, I would like to discuss the possibility of getting an initial few hours of unbroken sleep when the epidural is set up.
- I would like to discuss having the epidural wear off towards the end of labour so I can feel to push and change positions.
- If my baby's heart rate is reassuring and if it is appropriate, I would like to be intermittently monitored so I can move freely.
- I would prefer not to be disturbed when in active labour – please feel free to do any routine checks without asking for my permission.
- Please can we talk about the use of a warm compress for the second stage.
- I would like to be the first one to touch my baby and to lift them up to me, OR I would like my partner to do this.
- I would like to have skin-to-skin right away.
- If there is no medical emergency, we'd like weighing and measuring to wait so we can enjoy our first moments together as a family. 'No hatting, patting or chatting' please.
- I would like a physiological third stage, OR I would like active management of the third stage. My partner would/would not like to cut the cord, OR I would like to cut the cord.
- I would like help with breastfeeding right away/I am not planning on breastfeeding.
- We would like/not like our baby to have Vitamin K (injection or orally?).
- If my baby needs to be moved away from me I would like my partner to stay with them.

In the event of induction of labour, I would like:

- If appropriate, to have some time to walk about after having my waters broken to see if things get going by themselves before starting the synthetic oxytocin.

- To keep as active as possible and to be encouraged to do this and not be on the bed.
- To have any monitoring set up while I'm on the birth ball so I remain active.
- To have the IV for the synthetic oxytocin drip to be inserted in my non-dominant arm.
- To keep the lights low and interruptions to a minimum.
- To try without an epidural OR I would like an epidural.

In the event of an unplanned caesarean birth, if possible, I would like:

- To have our own music/hypnobirthing MP3s played throughout, if there is time for this.
- We would/would not like to be kept informed during the operation.
- To have the gown on back to front to enable skin-to-skin.
- To have any cannulas set up in my non-dominant hand and arm.
- To have skin-to-skin right away.
- To find out our baby's sex ourselves.
- To have the curtain lowered at the time of birth so I can see my baby being born.
- To wait at least one minute before the cord is clamped and cut.
- To bring our camera/phone in for first pictures.
- If my baby has to go to SCBU (special care baby unit), I want my partner to stay with them.

Remember the mother-centred caesarean birth mentioned in the caesarean birth chapter too – is this of interest? (This may be more likely in the event of a planned caesarean, as it would usually require discussion beforehand).

A reminder of things to consider in advance

- Whether or not you will consent to a membrane sweep.
- Your thoughts on your 'due date' – do you need to book in a chat with someone senior to personalise your plans?
- Do you need to think about a second birth partner/doula?
- Monitoring – what options are available to you?
- Whether or not you agree to having your waters released during

labour – also known as ARM (artificial rupture of membranes) or amniotomy – to speed up surges and make them stronger. This is not supported by evidence for women whose labours were spontaneous and are progressing normally, or if the labour has stalled. ARM can also make the surges feel stronger and more intense and may mean you now need to consider pain relief as a result.

Chapter twenty-two

Healing and resting after birth

→ In some parts of the world a real importance is placed on a period of healing, wellbeing and adjustment for a new mother. Often for many weeks a new mother is taken great care of, brought nourishing food and is kept away from busy day-to-day life with her baby close by.

In other parts of the world, and certainly here in the UK, this nurturing time of rest tends to get overlooked with women rushing to get back to normal after birth. This could be for many reasons of course – busy family life with other young children, not having family members or a support network close by, and so on – but also because perhaps getting 'back to normal' quickly is what she feels is expected of her.

Whatever type of birth you have had you need time to mentally adjust to becoming a mother, as well as time to physically heal. And of course partners need this time too! Days merge into nights and life feels very topsy-turvy as you get used to having a tiny baby 24/7. Therefore it is great to make a postnatal plan. While the birth is of course very important, so is your recovery.

Here are some ideas to think about before the baby arrives:

- Who can you call upon for general support for you once your baby is here?
- Who can come over who will take care of you? Who is a good listening ear who won't judge or talk over you or just be visiting to see the baby?
- What meals can you batch cook now so your freezer is well stocked with good, home-cooked food?
- Who do you trust enough to take your baby out for a walk and some fresh air to give you a little time alone?
- What favourite meals/foods do you want to have ready to eat when you get home? How about getting into bed with freshly changed sheets and snuggling with your baby, skin-to-skin, with all of your favourite foods next to you to eat in bed? Some women like to spend the first week in bed, then the second week on the sofa – then see how they feel after this.
- What local mother and baby groups are on in your area for whenever you feel ready for this sort of thing? There is no need to rush into attending these groups, but when you feel ready to do so it can feel great to talk to other parents! There may be some free meet-ups and walking groups – research now into what's out there.
- Maybe get an internet shop set up with a shopping list of all your favourites saved.

And on visitors...

- How do you feel about visitors after the birth? Would you prefer to have some time alone with your baby, just you and your partner, before welcoming visitors? Or are you happy to have visitors right away?
- Would you prefer to have everyone over on a set day, at a set time? How about asking them all to bring a dish so you can eat together? Get some paper plates/cups so you're not left with the washing up after they go.
- How about limiting visiting time? You could make it after lunch so it is clear that you are not providing a meal. Offer visiting from, say, 2–4pm – making it clear that after this you need to rest. Or you could say you will be in a pub/restaurant/wherever from 1–3pm and people can pop

by there to see the baby. Then you can leave when you've had enough and go back to an empty house.

- How useful will your visitors be? If they are the type who would nurture you by bringing food and some shopping and being mindful to leave when you're tired, then that's great.
- If you are planning on breastfeeding or wanting lots of skin-to-skin with your baby, it can be easier to sit with your top off spending time getting to grips with it all –this is perhaps less easy to do with a room full of relatives and visitors sitting around you.

Your baby may be over-stimulated by the inevitable 'pass the baby', and any strong perfumes or aftershaves people are wearing. Lying down in a dimly-lit room and having skin-to-skin can help to calm your baby. All they want is you, after all. Whatever you decide about visitors, sometimes it's best to let family and friends know your wishes now rather than when the baby is here and emotions are running high.

Bleeding after birth

Postnatal bleeding (lochia) is healthy and normal following any type of birth – both vaginal and caesarean – and is not painful, though some mothers experience 'after pains' when breastfeeding (less so with a first baby). If you are in pain speak to your midwife.

Lochia blood loss from the placental site continues until the lining is renewed. It can last up to six weeks, but it won't be heavy for all that time and many women find it gradually reduces and stops by around two weeks after the birth.

Stock up on around 3–4 packs of maternity pads for your hospital bag – do not use tampons. For the first day the blood loss is usually bright red and may have clots in it. If you are passing large clots (bigger than a 50p piece), lots of clots or are soaking through sanitary pads quickly, mention this to your midwife. Expect to change your pad around every 2–3 hours in the first few days.

Just like a period, the blood loss will change colour from red to a brown colour to a pinky mucous loss, becoming less and less over the first 10 days. For some women it peters out more quickly than for others. Once the loss has lessened you can use a panty liner rather than big, bulky maternity pads.

Stock up on large, comfortable cotton underwear – there is no need to buy throwaway paper underwear unless you want to.

Retained placenta

Sometimes a fragment of placenta may be left behind inside the uterus, which can cause problems and needs to be dealt with quickly. If you experience any of the following symptoms, go to your doctor or speak to your midwife.

- heavy bleeding
- cramping
- foul-smelling vaginal discharge
- fever
- a lack of breastmilk

Also contact your doctor if you have prolonged, heavy bleeding in the days or weeks following your baby's birth. Seek medical help if your blood flow peters out, then suddenly becomes very heavy again.

Pain relief after birth

Take advice from a qualified healthcare professional as to what types of painkillers are safe for you, as women's circumstances are varied.

Sex life

It is of course usual for your sex drive to take a back seat after birth! Adjusting to your new role and giving your body time to heal is important. Some women feel ready soon and others prefer to wait until their six-week check with the GP – or much longer.

Some women feel 'touched out' from holding, feeding and looking after a baby all day and all night, and this makes them less interested in getting intimate with their partner.

The type of birth you have will also have an impact on when you feel ready, and in what way. Stitches are usually all dissolved away by around 10 days after the birth – wait until any bleeding has stopped. An episiotomy will take longer to heal.

Be mindful that even if you're exclusively breastfeeding you can get pregnant before your period has restarted. At your six-week GP check your doctor will discuss safe methods of contraception, which may be different from your previous methods – for example, certain types of contraceptive pill may not be suitable if you are breastfeeding.

Emotions

Some parents feel a huge rush of love when they meet their baby for the first time, while for others it may take a little longer. Try not to worry if you don't feel strong love straight away. Many things can affect emotions and bonding with your baby, including how you and your partner feel your birth went. Go easy on yourself and give yourself time.

Having a baby can evoke a huge rollercoaster of emotions. It is normal for mothers to feel emotional, teary and overwhelmed after birth, without really knowing why they feel this way. Around 80 percent experience the so-called 'baby blues' at around day 4–5 after birth. No one really knows exactly what causes baby blues, but it is not an illness and usually passes within a few days or so. Symptoms include feeling irrational, teary, irritable, anxious or 'touchy'.

Sometimes parents feel depressed after the birth of their baby. It's not clear why some new parents experience depression and others do not.

Postnatal depression can affect both mothers and fathers. It can start at any time in the first year after your baby's birth, usually within six weeks, and can be mild or severe. Depression can be made worse by emotional and stressful events and what support a person has available has a huge effect on how they feel they can cope. How the birth went, along with disturbed sleep, any relationship issues, money pressures and so on can add to low feelings.

It's okay to have the odd day when you aren't enjoying parenthood or you don't feel like you're doing well at it. It's also normal to worry about your baby, or to have days where you feel down because it can feel very overwhelming to suddenly have responsibility for a baby. But you should also be having a lot of wonderful highs in among these feelings. If you feel like the lows are outweighing the highs, or you are being plagued with anxiety/anxious thoughts, do talk to someone.

Sometimes the person going through the depression is less aware and it may be loved ones who notice that the person has lost their spark, or seems very low.

The sooner your or your partner's feelings are talked through the better and you can do this with your GP or health visitor. Recovery may be slower for some than others, but it will happen. There is a lot of help out there (sources of help can be found at the end of the book) so reach out and use it if needed.

- Share your feelings with people you trust and who will not judge you. This could be a health visitor, a friend or a counsellor.
- Talking to other parents can be very reassuring, or those who have experienced postnatal depression before. There may be a local meet-up near you. There is also online support available.
- Try to get time away from your baby; even an hour here and there can make a difference.
- Take some exercise each day, such as a walk with your baby or perhaps doing a postnatal Pilates or yoga class. Exercise has a positive effect on mood.
- Maintain a healthy diet: eating badly or skipping meals can make you feel tired and irritable, so try to eat simple and nutritious meals.
- If you're feeling very low or wiped out, request a blood test to check iron levels, vitamin D levels, B12 levels and anything else the GP may suggest.
- Invest in a good quality multivitamin and eat as much fresh fruit and veg as you can.
- Accept help and support from family and friends.
- Give yourself time to adjust to parenthood.

Some parents worry that if they tell someone they are feeling depressed or that they are not bonding with their baby that their baby will be taken away from them. Your baby won't be taken away from you. Babies are only ever taken into care in very exceptional circumstances.

Postpartum psychosis

Postpartum psychosis (also known as puerperal psychosis) is a rare but serious mental illness which always requires psychiatric treatment and a stay in hospital. It only affects the mother, affecting around one or two mothers in every 1,000, and most commonly occurs in the first month after having a baby (usually within the first few days or so).

It's not known what causes postpartum psychosis, but a woman is more at risk if she already has a diagnosis of bipolar or schizophrenia or if there is a family history of postpartum psychosis.

The main symptoms are delusions, hallucinations, manic mood, feeling very confused, behaving in a way that's out of character and a lack of self-awareness. The person may not be aware they are unwell.

In very severe cases, a woman may try to harm her baby and/or herself, and medical help is required immediately and in the first instance via Accident & Emergency (A&E) who will then refer on for help with care going forward, or by calling 999. The most severe symptoms last 2–12 weeks, but it can take 6–12 months to fully recover, and a full recovery is very often made.

It's good to have a plan A, B and C in regards to your birth plan as already mentioned, but even with this in place, sometimes parents still feel disappointed that things didn't go the way they were hoping for.

Below are some ideas to think about should this occur:

- First off, know you did your very best! You did all you could at the time.
- Talk – find someone who will listen without interrupting. A good friend who can be a listening ear. It can really help to just offload your thoughts.
- Request your notes and go through these with a midwife/consultant midwife/obstetrician. You can arrange a debrief either with or without requesting your notes in advance.
- Speak to other mothers and join forums to know you are not alone.

You can self refer for free NHS therapy or counselling services, sometimes called talking therapies, via the IAPT (Improving Access to Psychological Therapies) or you can ask your GP to do this for you.

Nutrition

Even though your baby may sleep a lot in the day and evening, it is still surprisingly hard to fit in preparing and eating meals – unless you have planned in advance or have friends and family close by to help.

As already mentioned, you can prepare for this before the birth. For example, if you are making pasta sauce, cook for six instead of two and freeze four portions. Separate food into small dishes before freezing it, so that they can go directly into the oven without having to be defrosted first. Or make a vat of soup and bag and freeze several portions. Ask visitors to bring supplies (or even better a meal!).

There's no need to have any special diet after birth, though of course it goes without saying that plenty of fruits and vegetables and staying well hydrated is important.

Exercise

Gentle walks and pelvic floor exercises are safe to do as soon as you feel ready. Swimming is fine once postnatal bleeding has stopped. Unless you exercised regularly before the birth of your baby, it's usually best to start slowly and wait until your six-week postnatal check with your GP who can advise you before starting a serious exercise regime again. See this six-week sign off as giving you the go ahead to focus on strengthening your core and see an experienced postnatal Pilates instructor to help with this. This will be longer if you have had a caesarean birth, possibly three months or so – again be guided by your doctor. Be careful before embarking on jogging or high-impact exercise.

A mother and baby yoga or postnatal Pilates class would be great, as would getting out for some fresh air with your baby once a day for your all-important mental health.

You don't have to put up with leaking urine when you cough, sneeze or run. If possible, pay to see a women's health physio after six weeks who can check your pelvic floor and give you specific pelvic floor exercises that are best for you. You can get a referral via your GP, but waiting lists may be long.

End-of-session summary

- You've now looked at feeding your baby, how to put together a birth plan or list of birth preferences, and healing and recovery after birth.
- Perhaps you'd like to come up with a feeding plan and/or a postnatal plan with your partner and family/friends. What might your support network look like and, if relevant, what will happen once your partner is back at work?
- Now is the time to broach the idea of visitors in the early days with your family and friends if you have any strong views on this.
- Find out about mum and baby groups in your area that interest you, and what breastfeeding support there is.

Conclusion

$\rightarrow$ I hope this book has given you food for thought and faith in your incredible body and powerful mind. And I hope the suggested ideas for birth partners serve you well.

Remember the consultant midwife and know she is there to support you. Use her valuable expertise and get in touch to ask all the questions you want and to state your wishes for your birth. She will do her very best to work with you to help you to get the birth you are hoping for.

If you are being told 'You're not allowed to...' or 'You have to...' this is a sign that you need to ask more questions. Always take the time to do your own research and ensure you are getting personalised care.

While birth is unpredictable, there is so much you can do to make it a positive and empowering experience, even down to changing the labour ward room around.

If hypnobirthing is of interest, invest time and effort into practising this as soon as you can. Carve out time each day for a little breathing practice.

Remember, if you ask, it is usually possible for someone to take the time to explain things to you and possibly offer you a different option which hadn't been mentioned before. You deserve clear explanations on the benefits and risks of things being offered to you, and being pointed to evidence that backs this up to read in your own time.

If you don't ask you'll never know, and if you don't know your options you don't have any.

If you are pregnant and reading this book – know that you are built to do this and you are truly amazing.

I wish you all the very best for your birth and beyond. I love to hear from readers, so please do say hello via my Facebook page, Instagram or websites.

www.baby-bumps.net
www.innermedicine.co.uk
Instagram: baby_bumps_hypnobirthing
Facebook: www.facebook.com/HypnobirthingSouthLondon

Appendix

Hypnobirthing scripts

Disclaimer

Hypnosis is just as safe as meditation or guided relaxation and is generally very good for your mental and physical health. However, please do not participate if you have a history or diagnosis of psychosis, psychiatric issues, clinical depression or epilepsy, or you know of any other medical reason not to participate.

A simple rule of thumb is to check with your GP or doctor first if you have any medical or mental health conditions, or have had in the past, before listening to an MP3 or asking someone to read these scripts to you. Do not undertake hypnosis when under the influence of alcohol or drugs.

Only embark on any hypnosis practice when you are in a place where it is safe for you to relax and you do not need to be alert and aware of your immediate surroundings. After emerging from hypnosis give yourself some time to come back to the present and reorientate yourself before driving a car or operating any machinery.

MP3s of all these scripts can be accessed by typing this link into your internet browser: **www.baby-bumps.net/bookmp3s**. Alternatively, you or your partner could record the scripts on a phone or other device for you to listen to when you want to. Or your partner could simply read them aloud.

Script 1: Breathing practice and positive affirmations

It would be great if you could carve out around 10 minutes or so a day for breathing practice. Listening to this audio will help you to do that.

Remember not to be disheartened if you're unable to get very deep, long breaths at first. The more you practise, the easier it will get.

By the time you're ready to give birth your uterus will be very large, having expanded to many times its normal size. It is a super strong, powerful bag of muscle and, just like all muscles, for it to work well and with ease it needs a good oxygen supply and a good blood supply.

During labour you can help your uterus do its amazing job with slow, rhythmic breathing. Not only will this keep you feeling super calm and in control, it will also provide your uterus with all it needs to make each surge powerful and efficient.

It's all about the rhythm. Rhythmic breathing, rhythmic words, rhythmic movement.

Before we start, take a moment to scan your body and see if you can notice any tension being held anywhere. Now, take a deep breath in... and sigh or breathe any tension out. Make your whole body floppy and relaxed – like a puppet whose strings have all been released. This is a great way to greet each surge when you are in active labour.

One more time, take a deep breath in... and sigh or breathe out softly, effortlessly. Release all stress and tension easily.

Good. Let's try a few breathing techniques and ideas now. I'll talk you through each one before we try them out.

Counted breathing
In a moment, you're going to take a big breath in through your nose and softly sigh the breath out, trying to make the out-breath a little longer than the in-breath. Keep your shoulders relaxed and your jaw relaxed and loose. I will count out in for four and out for six, but if this feels too long or short for you adjust as you see fit and follow your own comfortable pattern of counting.

Beginning now. Breathing in, 2, 3, 4... and out 2...3...4...5...6...
And again - breathing in, 2, 3, 4... and out 2...3...4...5...6...
And now try two more breaths in and out, counting comfortably by yourself.

Visualisation using colour

Close your eyes and think of a colour that makes you feel calm and confident. Just pick the first colour that comes into your mind. Now you have that colour in your mind, keep your eyes closed and imagine that colour in front of you in all its vibrancy and beauty.

Now take a deep breath and inhale this strong, calm colour in through your nose. Fill your heart and lungs with this colour and feel it filling your belly now, swirling around your baby, soothing and calming your baby as it does so.

And when you're ready, now breathe out the colour, with a soft relaxed face and jaw, seeing the colour spreading far out in front of you, perhaps like when you're able to see your breath on a very cold day. The colour slowly drifts away from you, taking any tension along with it.

And again, let's do three more colour breaths – so you're going to breathe in the colour, a long, slow, deep breath, then sigh it out softly, seeing it drift away from you, taking all tension along with it.

Great. And the next breathing technique we're going to try is the rectangle visualisation.

Visualisation – rectangle

Now picture a rectangle in your mind's eye, or look at a door frame if there is one visible and you prefer to keep your eyes open. In a moment we're going to breathe in – 2, 3, 4 – on the short part of the rectangle, and out – 2, 3, 4, 5, 6 – on the longer part.

Let's start now – in your own time, complete three rectangle breaths.

Great. The next visualisation is the sea of strength, which I'll talk you through first.

Visualisation – sea of strength

In a moment you're going to picture yourself standing on a sea of strength, however you imagine this to look... Then you'll take a breath in, and as you do so feel the strength being drawn up through your feet, up your legs, into your torso, safely enveloping your baby, into your chest and neck and finally into your head, reviving you. And as you breathe out, imagine a shower of calm cascading down your head, body, all the way down to your toes, washing away any tension from your body and mind as it does so. Try this visualisation for three breaths now – in your own time breathing in strength on the in-breath, and feeling calm wash over you on your out-breaths.

Mantras

You can of course make your own up, but if you don't have any in mind, in a moment, try one of these while you practise three more slow, deep, calming breaths:

Beginning now. On the in-breath say 'I breathe in, I relax'... and on the out-breath say 'I breathe out, I am strong'....

And now on the in-breath, 'I breathe in, I am calm'.... and on the out-breath 'I breathe out, and I'm one step closer'...

And now on the in-breath say 'I breathe in strength'... and on the out-breath say 'I breathe out peace'.

And now 'I breathe in, I sink deeper, I breathe out, I float freely'.

Now try out three more breaths either with the mantras we just did, or words of your own choosing.

And finally, scan your body for any remaining tension. Take one last deep breath in, and on the out-breath try slowly saying relax, relax, relax – or any other word of your choice.

Great. I hope you're now feeling calm and relaxed.

Each day spend a few moments practising these breathing techniques. Try with your eyes closed, bringing your focus inwards, and with your eyes open as you're going about your day. It's also a lovely way to start and end the day and it is fantastic if birth partners can also do this practice.

Positive affirmations for labour and birth

I choose to feel good being me, I know I am capable.

I give birth easily and calmly.

My birth is smooth and comfortable.

I believe in my body and my baby.

Each breath and surge brings my baby closer to me.

Women all over the world are giving birth with me.

Breathing deeply and slowly relaxes my muscles, making my labour comfortable.

My body knows how to birth my baby, just as it knew how to grow my baby.

I am strong and I trust my body knows what to do.

I relax into each surge, maximising oxygen to me and my baby.

I keep gently active, I create space for my baby to be born swiftly and safely.

Surges are powerful and strong, but they are not stronger then me because they are me.

I am using my surges to birth my baby.

I relax and let my body take over, it knows what it's doing.

I breathe in relaxation, I breathe out softness.

As labour progresses my relaxation deepens and my body relaxes and opens.

Whatever turn my birth takes, I remain calm and in control.

I am able to make decisions about my birth clearly and calmly.

I am ready and looking forward to the birth of my baby.

Birth is a normal process

Birth is safe.

All is well.

Script 2: Safe place and confidence relaxation – mother

This script is written for the mother, with the birth partner's version to follow. I suggest listening to this early on, as you may find it useful to have a reference point for a 'safe place' during some of the other MP3s.

Just settle yourself into the most comfortable position and allow your eyes to gently close now... Allow yourself to settle more and more deeply into the chair or on the bed...

Now take a deep breath in.... and let it out slowly... and allow yourself to become more relaxed as you do so, as though you are breathing away all tensions from your mind and body... And allow your breathing to start to slow down and deepen...

And as you pause here for a moment you can let go of any unhelpful or unwanted thoughts... Just notice them and let them drift on by... For now, all you need to do is just relax and listen to my voice... Everything but my voice is fading into the background now... nothing else seems of interest... My voice is helping you to relax more and more, and to sink deeper and deeper and deeper into this wonderful feeling of relaxation... Just relax now... Relax.

Now I'm going to ask you to imagine it's a warm summer's day and you're in a wonderfully relaxing and pleasant place in nature, real or imagined... Just take a moment now to imagine this perfect place in nature... Imagine the feelings in your body... Notice how you breathe... Imagine that you can hear the sounds of that scene... as if you're there now, listening... Many people enjoy the sounds of nature, like the sound of a breeze among the trees, birds singing or waves rolling in and out... Even listen to the periods of silence between sounds...

Perhaps you'll notice the warmth of the sun on your skin?... Or the texture of things you touch along the way... Take a moment now to just relax and enjoy your peaceful surroundings...

Good. In a moment, I'm going to begin counting back from five down to zero. By the time I reach zero you will be right in the middle of that pleasant, relaxing scene, as if it's happening right now... Beginning now... Five, travelling deeper into the colours and the feelings... Four, getting deeper into that feeling... Three, getting deeper and deeper into those positive feelings... Two, almost there, you can imagine that scene so clearly... One... right there, right now... and on the count of zero, going right into the middle of that pleasant scene, deep into those good feelings, as if it's happening right now... Allow yourself to really believe that you're there, right now... Imagine what it feels like to know that you are safe and secure, to feel that you are relaxing completely into that scene...

Good.

You decide to walk around some more and further explore this beauty spot. And as you walk, with each step you allow your relaxation and feelings of safety to increase... As you continue to walk, relaxing more and more with each step, just take time to notice the things that interest you as you drift deeper and deeper into relaxation with each step you take...

You feel so peaceful, calm and comfortable in this place... This is your safe place... In this tranquil place nothing seems to bother you, you are just enjoying the quiet time here...

And in a moment you're going to find the perfect place to sit or lie *down and relax even more. Take a moment now to find the perfect spot...*

Now you've found an area to relax in you lean back and close your eyes, aware of the warmth of the sun...

As you close your eyes... you allow the wonderful warmth of the sun to relax and comfort your whole mind and body...

Notice as the warmth spreads all around the muscles of your eyes and eyelids... relaxing and soothing everything in its path... your cheeks, mouth and jaw muscles all begin to soften and relax... your tongue rests comfortably and relaxes... Notice as this lovely warmth now spreads down through your neck and shoulder muscles... you feel completely relaxed, comfortable and at peace... The comforting warmth moves down the length of your spine... releasing all tension, as you allow yourself to just let go...

Now the warmth gently moves down your arms, hands and fingers, as they become limp, relaxed and comfortable... you feel yourself starting to drift down into a feeling of deep relaxation and peace, as the warmth of the sun moves throughout your body... you feel safe as you know that this beautiful place is your safe place, just for you.

Now the warmth of the sun moves down the front of your body... bringing relaxation to your chest, stomach and pelvis, soothing and comforting you and your baby... you breathe calmness and peace down to your baby... Tune into your baby now for a moment or two, let them know that you can't wait to meet them and welcome them into the world... calmly and peacefully...

You feel confident and ready for the birth of your baby...

The gentle warmth of the sun moves down your legs now, relaxing and softening the muscles of your legs, feet and toes... as you move deeper and deeper into relaxation and peace... And now, your entire body is now bathed in soft, warm golden light... Relax, rest and do nothing.

You are now so deeply relaxed that your mind has become very receptive...

You do not need to learn how to give birth, your body already knows how to do this... When you feel your surges working you associate this with power and strength and you look forward to meeting your baby soon... When the time comes for your baby to begin their journey into the world, you are able to relax easily at home while in early labour...

And when it's time for you to leave home and go to hospital, or as you await the arrival of your home birth midwife, you feel just as you are sitting here now – totally relaxed and calm...

Your surges are powerful – but you know they are nothing more than muscles working hard to bring your baby safely to you... a normal physiological function... And so you welcome each one, using them as a signal to go much deeper into relaxation.

You will be doing hard work, but you've done hard work before and you are capable... There may be times when you feel an intensity like you've never felt before, but this does not surprise you or worry you because you know this is perfectly normal... Instead you notice how easily your mind eases the pressure, letting it spread and flow and dissipate...

You are preparing for all of this ahead of time, training your nervous system to relax so that no matter what eventuality or situation may occur, no matter whether there are delays or surprises, you know you have the freedom to choose to trust and relax... You are always in control...

You use each surge to go deeper into relaxation and trust... each one brings you closer and closer to holding your baby in your arms... Birth is generally very safe indeed and you are in safe hands, you have the knowledge of countless women with you...

All you need to do is relax and let your body take over, busy doing its own work...

You easily distract yourself and when you feel a surge begin, without thinking, you relax deeper into hypnosis, and you remain there for as long as the surge lasts.

You know that during a surge you can slowly count down from five to zero and when you reach zero you will be completely relaxed... five, four, three, two, one, zero and relax...

As soon as each surge finishes this means it's completed and can be forgotten. You get to relax in between each surge...

Throughout your whole labour, should you need to open your eyes, talk or answer any questions you will be able to do so while remaining deep in hypnotic relaxation... Any noises you hear from others inside or outside of the room will not disturb you – instead they are a signal for you to deepen your hypnosis and comfort. Any negative talk in the room becomes white noise to you and just allows you to go deeper into relaxation...

Every time you listen to this relaxation you find that you relax more and more quickly, easily and deeply. The suggestions become more and more a part of you... They are working more effectively than you can possibly imagine...

Now you are feeling relaxed, confident and calm you can create a cue for these feelings of trust by placing your right hand on your left shoulder. And any time you want to feel as calm and relaxed as you do now just close your eyes, place your right hand on your left shoulder and take a deep breath in. On the out-breath breathe out any tension, letting your right hand sink all the way to your side, bringing about deep relaxation. This cue is a signal to go deeper and deeper into trust and relaxation... And again, place your hand on your shoulder, breathe in, and on the relaxing out-breath let your hand slide all the way down your arm... One more time... place your hand on your shoulder, breathe in and on the out-breath let your arms slide all the way down. This cue also works when your partner or midwife puts a hand on your shoulder.

Good. And so, in a moment or two it will be time to come back to the present knowing you can return to your safe place and recover all these good feelings anytime you choose to... Just imagining it makes you feel good, and those feelings come much more easily to mind now, and perhaps you can even imagine that safe place and those good feelings are always there, all of the time, at the back of your mind somewhere. There's always a part of you which already knows those positive feelings completely... And you can take as much of those good feelings with you as you want right now...

And now I'm going to count from one to five and when I get to five you will be wide awake and alert, feeling relaxed, refreshed and ready to continue with your day...

If you would like to drift off into a restful, deep sleep, then this is absolutely fine... you will wake up feeling refreshed and relaxed...

Beginning now.

One, starting to become more aware of your body where you are sitting. Two, picturing the room around you now. Three, your eyelids are becoming lighter. Four, feeling more awake and alert. Five, opening your eyes now, completely out of hypnosis, alert, refreshed and ready to continue with your day.

Script 3: Safe place and confidence relaxation - birth partner

This script is for the birth partner. He or she can listen to this a few times a week, or once a day if the due date is close.

Just settle yourself into the most comfortable position and allow your eyes to gently close now. Allow yourself to settle more and more deeply into the chair or on the bed...

Now take a deep breath in... and let it out slowly... and allow yourself to become more relaxed as you do so... as though you are breathing away all tensions from your mind and body...

Now bring your attention to your breathing and allow your breathing to start to slow down and deepen...

And as you pause here for a moment, let go of all unhelpful or unwanted thoughts... Any thoughts that come into your mind you allow to float on by... For now, just relax and listen to my voice. Everything but my voice is fading into the background now, nothing else seems of interest... My voice is helping you to relax more and more and to sink deeper and deeper and deeper into this wonderful feeling of relaxation... Just relax now... Relax...

And now, imagine it's a warm summer's day and you're in a wonderfully relaxing and pleasant place in nature, real or imagined. Just take a moment now to imagine this perfect place in nature... Imagine how relaxed your body feels... Notice how you breathe... Imagine that you can hear the sounds of that scene... as if you're there now, listening... Many people enjoy the sounds of nature, like the sound of a breeze among the trees, birds singing or waves rolling in and out... Even listen to the periods of silence between sounds...

Perhaps you'll notice the warmth of the sun on your skin... Or the texture of things you touch along the way... Take a moment now to just relax and enjoy your peaceful surroundings...

Good. In a moment, I'm going to begin counting back from five down to zero, and by the time I reach zero you will be right in the middle of that pleasant, relaxing scene, as if it's happening right now... Beginning now... Five, travelling deeper into the colours and the feelings... Four, getting deeper into that feeling... Three, getting deeper and deeper into those positive feelings... Two, almost there, you can imagine that scene clearly... One... right there, right now... and on the count of zero, going right into the middle of that pleasant scene, deep into those good feelings, as if it's happening right now... Allow yourself to really believe that you're there, right now... Imagine what it feels like to know that you are safe and secure, to feel that you are relaxing completely into that scene... Imagine the feelings in your body... Notice how you breathe... Good.

You decide to walk around some more and further explore this beauty spot... And as you walk with each step you allow your relaxation to increase... As you continue to walk, relaxing more and more with each step, just take time to notice the things that interest you as you drift deeper and deeper into relaxation with each step you take...

You feel so peaceful, calm and comfortable in this place... This is your safe place, in this tranquil place nothing seems to bother you, you are just enjoying the quiet time here...

And in a moment you're going to find the perfect place to sit or lie down and relax even more. Take a moment now to find the perfect spot...

Now you've found an area to relax in you lean back and close your eyes, aware of the warmth of the sun...

As you close your eyes... you allow the wonderful warmth of the sun to relax and comfort your whole mind and body...

Notice as the warmth spreads all around the muscles of your eyes and eyelids... relaxing and soothing everything in its path... your cheeks, mouth and jaw muscles all begin to soften and relax... your tongue rests comfortably in your mouth... notice as this lovely warmth now spreads down through your neck and shoulder muscles... you feel completely relaxed, comfortable and at peace... as the comforting warmth moves down the length of your spine... releasing all tension, as you allow yourself to let go and relax...

Now the warmth gently moves down your arms, hands and fingers, as they become limp, relaxed and comfortable... you feel yourself starting to drift down into a feeling of deep relaxation and peace, as the warmth of the sun moves throughout your body... you feel safe as you know that this beautiful place is your safe place, just for you...

Now the warmth of the sun moves down the front of your body... bringing relaxation to your chest, stomach and pelvis...

You feel confident and ready to support your partner during your baby's birth...

The gentle warmth of the sun moves down your legs now, relaxing and softening the muscles of your legs, feet and toes... as you move deeper and deeper into relaxation and peace... your entire body is now bathed in soft, warm golden light... Relax, rest and do nothing...

You are now so deeply relaxed that your mind has become very receptive...

When the time comes for your baby to begin their journey into the world, you are able to relax easily at home in the early stages, knowing exactly how best to support your partner at this exciting time, encouraging her to both rest and be gently active... You feel calm and confident in your supportive role...

And, when the time comes for you to leave home and go to hospital, or as you await the arrival of your home birth midwife, you feel just as you are sitting here now – totally relaxed and calm...

And when your partner's labour intensifies you know exactly how best to comfort her. You remember everything you have learned... You remain calm as your partner's surges intensify... You know your partner's powerful surges are nothing more than her muscles working hard to bring your baby safely into the world, they are a normal physiological function...

You are preparing for all of this ahead of time, training your nervous system to relax so that no matter what eventuality or situation may occur, no matter whether there are delays or surprises, you know you have the freedom to choose to trust in the process and relax... You are always in control and you always know how best to support your partner...

You are able to communicate with the midwives and doctors with ease, remembering all that you want to ask, easily gathering the information needed to, along with your caregivers, help you and your partner make any decisions that are required...

Birth is generally very safe indeed and your partner is in safe hands...

In the unlikely event you feel you are starting to not think straight, you quickly and easily distract yourself, reminding yourself that you are clear-headed and calm and that you know your partner best... You know how best to support her, better than anyone else...

You know that you can use the technique of taking a big breath in and slowly counting down on the out-breath from five to zero. You know when you reach zero you will be completely relaxed and clear-headed... five, four, three, two, one, zero and relax... Relax now...

Every time you listen to this relaxation you find that you relax *more and more quickly, easily and deeply. The suggestions become more and more a part of you. They are working more effectively than you can possibly imagine...*

Now you are feeling relaxed, confident and calm you can create a cue for these good feelings of trust by placing your thumb and finger together. And any time you want to feel as calm and relaxed as you do right now, just take a deep breath in, breathe out, relax... and bring your thumb and finger together... And again, breathing in, and on the out-breath, relax and bring your thumb and finger together... One more time, breathing in, and on the out-breath bring your thumb and finger together...

Good. And so, in a moment or two, it will be time to come back to the present knowing you can return to your safe place and recover all these good feelings of confidence and trust anytime you choose to do so. Just imagining it makes you feel good, and those feelings come much more easily to mind now, and perhaps you can even imagine that safe place and those good feelings are always there, all of the time, at the back of your mind somewhere, there's always a part of you which already knows those positive feelings completely... And you can take as much of those good feelings with you as you want right now.

And now I'm going to count from one to five and when I get to the number five you will be wide awake and alert, feeling relaxed, refreshed and ready to continue with your day...

If instead you would like to drift off into a restful, deep sleep, then this is absolutely fine... you will wake up feeling refreshed and relaxed...

Beginning now.

One, starting to become more aware of your body where you are sitting. Two, picturing the room around you now. Three, your eyelids are becoming lighter. Four, feeling more awake and alert. Five, opening your eyes now, completely out of hypnosis, alert, refreshed and ready to continue with your day.

Script 4: Fear-release script

You can listen to this comforting track any time, but it may be especially useful if you are having a day where you're feeling anxious or worried about your upcoming birth.

I'd like you to get comfortable, take a moment and make sure you're happy with your posture, feet flat on the floor... rest comfortably and close your eyes... Allow your breathing to slow down and become relaxed and smooth... As you breathe, in... and out... you're starting to feel your body relax and sink comfortably down. Any external sounds you hear or any sensations you feel simply help you to go deeper into relaxation and hypnosis.

And now, in your own time, take three deep, slow breaths in... and out... and with each out-breath you start to feel any tension dropping away...

Now that you're beginning to relax we can focus on deepening this relaxation further, throughout your entire body... Beginning now. Slowly bring your attention to the soles of your feet and imagine this feeling of relaxation spreading over your feet, dissolving tension from all the muscles as it does so... Now it flows all the way over your ankles and up through both legs... send that feeling up through your calves now, your shins and into your knees... and let the lower part of your legs relax completely. Now imagine that feeling rising up through your thighs and into the hips and pelvis... imagine both legs relaxing over and over again... Now imagine that feeling spreading up into your abdomen... into the waist and up through your torso... Imagine that feeling of deep relaxation spreading up into your chest and shoulders... up over the shoulders and down into the arms... Let your shoulders sink comfortably down and your arms loosen, relax and hang limp and heavy... Allow your breathing to become slow and rhythmic... effortless... Now imagine that sense of relaxation spreading from the base of the spine all the way up each part of your back in turn... each segment of your spine, right up to the nape of your neck... Let the sensation flow over the back of your head, over your scalp and down over your forehead... Relax all the muscles in and around your eyes... Let this feeling of peace and relaxation spread over your cheeks and down your jaw... Send these relaxing feelings into your mouth, soften all the muscles in the mouth and relax your jaw. Let your tongue relax. Your whole face has a completely relaxed expression, as if you are in a deep sleep.

Pause for a moment and scan your face and body – if you note any areas of tension that may have crept back in, release it all gently now on your next out-breath... Every last bit of tension is now draining out of your body and mind so you can enjoy this restful feeling... Rest and relax and do nothing...

Good. Now I'd like you to picture something like a volume slider with the numbers three to zero on it. In a moment we're going to enjoy three slow, calming breaths and as you release tension on each out-breath you see the slider moving towards the zero... from three down to two and then two down to one and finally one down to zero, helping you to sink down further into relaxation. So go ahead and take three breaths in and out, allowing your relaxation to easily deepen with each out-breath... Now you are on zero and are very relaxed indeed. And again, zero. Deeply relaxed... Just enjoy this feeling for a moment or two...

Now that you are feeling calm and at ease, I am going to talk you through a gentle, guided relaxation. If you notice your mind wandering during the relaxation just gently guide it back to my voice.

Any sounds that break in, such as voices outside or cars passing by, will just send you into a deeper relaxation, so just let these sounds drift on through you...

I want you to use your imagination and see yourself walking towards a beautiful beach. It can be a beach you know, or it can be an imagined beach...

It's a lovely day and the temperature is just right... Feel the warm breeze gently blowing across your face and skin... Breathe in and smell the fresh sea air...

This area is completely safe, and, apart from a few people far away in the distance, it's just you here.

You walk down a pathway leading to the soft sandy beach. You are enjoying the quietness of the beach. You can hear the gentle, rhythmic sound of the waves rolling in... and out... Such a calm and lovely place to be.

You arrive at some steps leading down to the beach. You take off your shoes and feel the warm, sandy steps beneath your bare feet... There are ten steps down, and as I count them, with each step down you feel more and more and more relaxed.

Ten... Nine... pausing for a moment, breathing deeply... smelling *the sea air... feeling relaxed... Eight... Seven... you feel your feet on the warm steps... notice how relaxed you now feel. Six... Five... each step down brings with it more relaxation... Four... Three... your relaxation is becoming deeper and deeper... Two... you feel so relaxed, comfortable and at peace... One and zero, you are now on the beach, feet sinking into the warm sand, feeling so good.*

You decide to walk down to the water's edge. You watch the soft waves rolling into the shore... You breathe in the fresh sea air... You look out over the water, far into the horizon... The clear blue sky looks beautiful against the green-blue sea... This wonderful place always makes you feel totally relaxed and at ease...

Now imagine yourself walking a short way away from the shore onto the warm sandy beach where you lay out your towel and drop your shoes onto the sand, and sit down...

Next to you is a small wooden boat with a rope attached to the front. This is a special boat which has the capacity to take away all worries and concerns...

Pause for a moment now, and consider any concerns you have, these could be about labour, birth or anything at all that is worrying you...

And now, taking your time, see yourself either mentally or physically putting each and every one of these worries or concerns into the little wooden boat... However you imagine each worry, I want you to see yourself putting each one inside the boat. It could be words, images or just mentally imagining it... Take a few moments now and pile all of the worries into the boat feeling lighter and lighter as each worry leaves your body and mind...

Now that all of your worries are piled in the small, light wooden boat, you stand up, pick up the rope and pull the boat the few steps towards the shore...

Now you're at the edge of the shore, you give the boat a firm push into the sea. The current takes the boat out into the sea... You watch the boat drift further... and further away... The boat with all your worries inside it becomes smaller and smaller and smaller, until it is a tiny dot in the distance... and then it completely disappears from your sight, taking all your concerns with it, each and every worry gone forever...

Standing at the shore, you take a deep breath in... and out.... and you feel so light and free, happy and relaxed...

Enjoying your new worry-free self you walk back to your towel, lie down comfortably and feel the warm rays of the glorious sunshine on your skin.

The warm sunshine and the rhythmic sound of the waves makes you feel even more drowsy and relaxed – in fact you are feeling more relaxed and peaceful than you have for a very long time...

Now, as you lie comfortably down, take a moment to imagine, seeing everything through your own eyes, how calm and relaxed your baby's birth will be... who will be there supporting you... where you will be, and how confident and at ease you will feel...

And now focus on your baby's arrival and, through your own eyes, see you both together, everything went as you hoped for. The atmosphere is calm and your baby is in your arms... Feel your baby's heavy, warm weight in your arms... You are so happy and content that everything went just as you visualised it... And this imagery is taking root deep within your mind, permanently and positively...

So it's now time to leave the beach, feeling assured, light and free of worry. You know this confidence and relaxation that you have created is here to stay with you throughout your pregnancy, your baby's birth and beyond...

You love how confident you feel. So calm, so rested, so energised...

You feel strong and in control. You are capable. You know all is well...

If you have fallen asleep and have no need to wake up, just continue your restful sleep. Should you need to get up and continue with your day you can now start walking back towards the steps.

I will now count your steps back up. As I count you are emerging from hypnosis. Feeling good... With each number I count your confidence grows... On the tenth step you will come back to the present feeling excited, confident and so ready for your baby's birth.

Beginning now. One, two three, feeling the energy in your arms and legs. Four, five, six, you're becoming more aware of the room around you. Seven and eight, you take a deep breath in and feel yourself becoming more alert. Nine, you are now coming back to the present time feeling happy and knowing all is well. And ten, you open your eyes, emerging completely from hypnosis, feeling alert, calm and refreshed.

Script 5: Top-to-toe tension release/Pre-surge body scan

This is a lovely script to listen to as part of your daily breathing exercises. Practising this longer tension release now will help you be able to do a quicker, more efficient pre-surge body scan. Let your partner know which word you chose at the end of the relaxation so they know what it is and you can let them know when it might help to say it to you – perhaps at the beginning or end of a surge.

Begin by closing your eyes and gently bring your attention to your breathing. Don't try to alter it, just pay attention to it for a moment...

Now focus on your physical body – where are you feeling tension or tightness? Again, just notice where it is held in your body for now...

In a moment we are going to start to release all tension from your body, using your breath. Bringing soothing relaxation to you on the in-breath and releasing any tension on the out-breath. During the relaxation simply follow your own comfortable breathing pattern so nothing feels forced. There will be time for you to do two relaxing breaths for each body section if you wish to – just take your second breath in whenever you need to. Breathe normally in between the sections.

If your mind wanders throughout this relaxation, just bring it back to your breath and the body part you want to focus on.

Beginning now. Make yourself comfortable... Close your eyes... Let your whole body start to relax as deeply as possible... Make no effort at all... Just imagine your body hanging loose, like a puppet whose strings have all been released... All your muscles limp, loose and comfortable.

Now, focus on the top of your head. Take a slow easy breath in and, on the out-breath, send a wave of relaxation over the top of your head, relaxing down into your forehead and down the back of your head into the nape of your neck... Then repeat this, with another breath in your own time...

Now focus on your eyes and the lower part of your face. Breathe in, and on the out-breath relax all the muscles in and around your eyes... Let this wonderful feeling of relaxation spread over your cheeks and down your jaw. Send these relaxing feelings into your mouth, soften all the muscles in the mouth and jaw. Let your tongue relax... And again, whenever you're ready...

Good.

Now focus on your neck and shoulders. Breathe in, and let the out-breath carry away any stress and tightness you have in these areas... All tension releasing as your shoulders heavily and naturally sink down on your next two out-breaths...

Bring your attention to your arms and hands now. Breathe in, and on the out-breath feel your arms becoming heavy and limp – all tension releasing down your arms and out through your fingertips. Let your shoulders sink comfortably down and your arms loosen, relax and hang limp and heavy...

Now it's time to relax your back. Breathe in and on the out-breath allow the relaxation to spread from your neck down into the top of your spine all the way down each part of your back in turn. Each segment of your spine is now releasing and relaxing...

I wonder if you're starting to notice that you now feel very relaxed. Feeling super-relaxed and peaceful.

And your breathing is slow and rhythmic.

Good. Now focus on your stomach and mid-lower back. Tune into your baby – whether they are active or sleeping, he or she is enjoying this wonderful calmness you're giving them. Spend time now relaxing these areas, sending love to your baby and feel yourself drifting into a deep relaxation with the next two out-breaths...

And now your bottom, pelvis and hips. Let go of any tightness and tension held here with your out-breath, sigh it all out...

And finally, your legs all the way down to your toes. Breathe in, and on the out-breath enjoy this feeling of relaxation spreading over the tops of your legs, the backs of your legs, down your thighs, into your knees and your calves, dissolving tension from the muscles as it does. Now it flows all the way over your ankles into your feet. Imagine both legs relaxing over and over again...

Good.

Your body is now relaxed from head to toe. Rest, relax and do nothing...

If you want to, you can think of a word which represents this relaxation that you have just created. It could be 'calm', 'relax', 'peace', 'safe' 'release'... or something else. Whatever word you decide on just repeat it to yourself in your head or out loud for a moment now...

Now place your thumb and finger together to create a cue to generate these feelings of relaxation and confidence... Along with your chosen word you can use this as a signal to go deeper into trust, confidence and relaxation... So breathe in, and on the relaxing out-breath place your thumb and finger together... and again, breathing in, and on the out-breath bring your thumb and finger together, perhaps while saying your chosen word... One more time, breathe in, and on the out-breath use your cue of bringing your thumb and finger together as you enjoy these feelings of relaxation and confidence... Good. Any time you want these good feelings to easily return you can use this cue, with or without your chosen word...

You are growing your baby perfectly, he or she is carefully preparing to enter this world with calm relaxation... Birth is a normal process... You constantly remind yourself of how strong and courageous you are. You easily adjust to whatever environment you find yourself in... You do everything better when you are relaxed... You can control your entire body with your mind... You are relaxed and strong. You know you are relaxed and strong...

And now it's time to come back to the present... If you've fallen asleep and have no need to get up, enjoy a deep, restful sleep. Otherwise I will count from one to five and on the number five you will be wide awake and alert, feeling good.

Beginning now. One, slowly become aware of your fingers and toes... two, becoming more aware of the room around you. Three, your eyelids are starting to feel lighter. Four, feeling the weight of your body fully now... and five, slowly opening your eyes. Eyes open, feeling refreshed, alert and keeping this relaxation with you for the rest of the day.

Script 6: Caesarean birth

This script is for those women who are having a planned caesarean birth, or whose circumstances have changed and will now be having their baby by caesarean.

Just settle yourself into the most comfortable position and gently close your eyes now... Allow yourself to settle more and more deeply into the chair or on the bed...

Now take a deep breath in... and let it out slowly... and allow yourself to become more relaxed as you do so... as though you are breathing away all tensions from your mind and body...

Now bring your attention to your breathing and let your breathing start to slow down and deepen...

And as you pause here for a moment you can allow any unwanted or unhelpful thoughts to drift on by... Dissolve away... For now just relax and listen to my voice... Everything but my voice is fading away now, nothing else seems of interest... My voice is helping you to relax more and more and to sink deeper and deeper and deeper into this wonderful feeling of relaxation... Just relax now. Relax...

Now you're starting to relax we can focus on deepening this relaxation further, through your entire body... Begin by bringing your attention to the soles of your feet and imagine this feeling of relaxation spreading over your feet, dissolving tension from the muscles as it does... Now it flows all the way over your ankles and up through your legs... send that feeling up through your calves, shins and into the knees and let the lower part of your legs relax completely... Now imagine that feeling rising up through the thighs and the backs of your legs and into your hips and pelvis... imagine both legs relaxing over and over again... Now imagine that feeling spreading up into the abdomen, the waist and up through your torso... Imagine that feeling spreading up into your chest and shoulders, up over the shoulders and down into your arms... Let your shoulders sink comfortably down and your arms loosen, relax and hang limp and heavy... Allow your breathing to become slow and rhythmic, effortless... Now imagine that sense of relaxation spreading from the base of the spine all the way up each part of your back in turn... each segment of your spine... right up to the nape of your neck... Let the sensation flow over the back of your head, over your scalp and down over your forehead... Relax all the muscles in and around your eyes. Let the feeling spread over your cheeks and down your jaw. Send these relaxing feelings into your mouth, soften all the muscles in the mouth and jaw. Let your tongue relax, resting comfortably. Your whole face has a completely relaxed expression, as if you are in a deep sleep.

Pause for a moment and scan your face and body – if you note any areas of tension that may have crept back in, release it all gently now on your next out breath... Every last bit of tension is now draining out of your body and mind so you can enjoy this restful feeling... Rest, relax and do nothing...

Now I'd like you to picture something like a volume slider with the numbers three to zero on it. In a moment we're going to enjoy three slow, calming breaths, and as you release tension on each out breath you see the slider turn down from three to two, then two to one, and finally one to zero, helping you to sink down further into hypnosis. So go ahead and take three breaths in and out, allowing your relaxation to easily deepen with each out-breath... Now you are on zero and are very relaxed indeed. And again, zero. Deeply relaxed and open to all positive suggestion.

Your entire body feels heavy, warm, soft and completely free of tension. Just enjoy this feeling for a moment or two...

Now that you are feeling calm and at ease, you are going to listen to some pleasant, relaxing hypnotic suggestions. If you notice your mind wandering during the relaxation just gently guide it back to my voice... Any sounds you hear, such as voices outside or cars passing by, will just send you deeper into hypnosis, so just let these sounds drift on through you...

For whatever reasons which are personal to you and right for you and your baby, you are going to give birth by caesarean. Your baby's birth will be peaceful and calm. You are at peace with your decision.

You know you will be in very good hands. In fact, you could not be in better hands. You will find that everything will go perfectly, smoothly... and you find you relax easily throughout. It's much easier to relax than most people ever realise...

The night before your baby's birth you will enjoy a restful sleep and will awake with feelings of calm anticipation, looking forward to meeting your baby...

When you arrive at hospital you can just ignore all the goings-on in the hospital, ignore the noise and the lights, ignore the chatting and general busyness... Nothing bothers you... You relax into your new surroundings with confidence and ease...

And from the moment the first medication or procedure is given to you, you relax as you know this is a signal for you to start to go to your safe place of confidence and trust... This place of confidence and trust may already be very familiar to you, but if not, that doesn't matter as you are now easily able to imagine a place where you feel safe and at ease... Perhaps this is a place in nature, or a particular room in a house... Take a moment now to go right to that place and notice what you see... Just relax in that safe place and enjoy it for a moment now... Good.

And when it's time to go to theatre you do so with happy excitement. Finally, the moment has come when you will meet your baby! You are calm and prepared... You meet the experienced team who will take great care of you and all you notice is a sea of welcoming, smiling faces, everything else blurs into insignificance...

During the procedure if you want to you can just close your eyes and go within... You can focus on your breathing and go to your safe place... You are pleasantly surprised at how easy it is to let all noise and activity around you fade away into the background... Notice how pleasant it is to know you don't need to bother to respond to anything at all, unless it is directed specifically to you...

You may notice how easy it is to tune into the smooth rhythm of your relaxed breathing... As you inhale... and exhale... your chest rises and falls in a comfortable easy rhythm... And each time you exhale you relax a little more, sinking deeply into the bed you are on, heavy, loose and limp... Your heartbeat is regular and even throughout your baby's birth... You relax knowing you are in safe hands and that you are going to meet your baby very, very soon...

And now, even more quickly than you imagined was possible, your baby is here, placed safely in your arms... Everything went perfectly and you are both doing very well... The healing process has already begun and your immune system is working at full speed to help you to recover quickly and easily...

You transfer to the recovery area and then eventually to the postnatal ward and you are relaxed and comfortable... You are pleased to find that you can move about quite well... You feel good, knowing all is well and you trust your body to heal quickly... All bodily functions return to normal rapidly as the anaesthetic wears off and you feel comfortable...

And now, you are home, safely tucked up in bed with your baby by your side... You are so relaxed and happy. Just enjoy this moment for a while now, enjoy the relief you feel and the joy that your baby is finally here, and you are both home, safe and sound... Now you can look forward to getting better fast and enjoying your beautiful baby... Just relax, rest and do nothing...

Now bring your thumb and finger together to create a cue for these happy, relaxed feelings and any time you want to feel as calm and relaxed as you do now just close your eyes, take a deep breath in and bring your thumb and finger together while breathing out any tension. And again, breathe in, and on the out-breath bring your finger and thumb together... One more time, breathing in, relax on the out-breath, bringing your thumb and finger together. Good...

Every time you listen to this relaxation you find that you relax more and more quickly, easily and deeply. The suggestions become more and more a part of you. They are working more effectively than you can possibly imagine.

And so in a moment or two it will be time to come back to the present knowing you are well prepared for your baby's birth. Bringing all these good feelings of confidence and trust in the staff, in the process and in your decision deep within you, giving you a feeling of peace and calm... knowing you can bring about all these good feelings anytime you choose to do so... And these good feelings come much more easily to mind now every time you think of your upcoming birth... And you can take as much of those good feelings with you as you want to right now.

And now I'm going to count from one to five and when I get to the number five you will be wide awake and alert, feeling relaxed, refreshed and ready to continue with your day...

If instead you would like to drift off into a restful, deep sleep, then this is absolutely fine... you will wake up feeling refreshed and relaxed...

Beginning now.

One, starting to become more aware of your body... your fingers, your toes... Two, picturing the room around you now. Three, your eyelids are becoming lighter. Four, feeling more awake and alert. Five, opening your eyes now, completely out of hypnosis, alert, refreshed and ready to continue with your day.

Script 7: Induction of labour

This script is for women who will be having an induction of labour.

Just settle yourself into the most comfortable position and allow your eyes to gently close now. Allow yourself to settle more and more deeply into the chair or wherever you are sitting...

Now take a deep breath in... and let it out slowly... and allow yourself to become more relaxed as you do so... as though you are breathing away all tensions from your mind and body.

Now bring your attention to your breathing and allow your breathing to start to slow down and deepen.

And as you pause here for a moment you allow all unhelpful or unwanted thoughts to drift on by... To dissolve away... For now just relax and listen to my voice. Everything but my voice is fading into the background, nothing else seems of interest. My voice is helping you to relax more and more and to sink deeper and deeper and deeper into this wonderful feeling of relaxation. Just relax now. Relax.

Now you're starting to relax we can focus on deepening this hypnotic relaxation further, through your entire body... Beginning now. Focus on the soles of your feet and imagine this feeling of relaxation spreading over your feet, dissolving tension from the muscles as it does. Now it flows all the way over the ankles and up through the legs. Send that feeling up through the calves, shins and into the knees and let the lower part of your legs relax completely. Now imagine that feeling rising up through the thighs and into the hips and pelvis, imagine both legs relaxing over and over again. Now imagine that feeling spreading up into the abdomen, into the waist and up through your torso. Imagine that feeling spreading up into your chest and shoulders, up over the shoulders and down into the arms. Let your shoulders sink comfortably down and your arms loosen, relax and hang limp and heavy. Allow your breathing to become slow and rhythmic, effortless. Now imagine that sense of relaxation spreading from the base of the spine all the way up each part of your back in turn, each segment of your spine, right up to the nape of your neck. Let the sensation flow over the back of your head, over your scalp and down over your forehead. Relax all the muscles in and around your eyes. Let the feeling spread over your cheeks and down your jaw. Send these relaxing feelings into your mouth, soften all the muscles in the mouth and jaw. Let your tongue relax, resting comfortably in your mouth. Your whole face has a completely relaxed expression, as if you are in a deep sleep.

Pause for a moment and scan your face and body – if you note any areas of tension that may have crept back in, release it all gently now on your next out-breath. Every last bit of tension is now draining out of your body and mind so you can enjoy this restful feeling. Rest, relax and do nothing.

Now I'd like you to picture a volume slider with the numbers three to zero on it. In a moment we're going to enjoy three slow, calming breaths and as you release tension on the out-breath you see the slider go from three to two, then two to one, and finally one to zero, helping you to sink down further into hypnosis. So go ahead and take three breaths in and out, allowing your relaxation to easily deepen with each out-breath... Now you are on zero and are very relaxed indeed. And again, zero. Deeply relaxed.

Your entire body feels heavy, warm, soft and completely free of tension. Just enjoy this feeling for a moment or two...

Now that you are feeling calm and at ease, I am going to talk you through a gentle, guided relaxation. If you notice your mind wandering during the relaxation just gently guide it back to my voice.

Any sounds that break in, such as voices outside or cars passing by, will just send you deeper into hypnosis, so just let any sounds drift on through you.

For whatever reasons which are personal to you and right for you and your baby, you have agreed to an induction of labour. Your baby's birth will be calm and peaceful. You are at peace with your decision.

In advance of your baby's birth you will find that you are able to gather any information needed to help you make informed decisions that are right for you... You will also be able to make decisions during your baby's birth, while remaining in hypnosis. Everything will go smoothly... and you find you relax easily throughout. It's much easier to relax than most people ever realise...

The night before you go in for your induction you will enjoy a restful sleep and will awake with feelings of calm anticipation, looking forward to meeting your baby.

When you arrive at hospital you can just ignore all the goings-on in the hospital, ignore the noise and the lights, ignore the chatting and general busyness. Nothing bothers you. You relax into your new surroundings with confidence and ease. There may be lots of waiting around, but you find the time passes quickly and you are able to keep your oxytocin levels high and your adrenalin levels low in all the ways which you know best.

And from the moment the first medication or procedure is given to you, you relax as you know this is a signal for you to start to go to your safe place of confidence and trust... Take a moment now to imagine your safe place of confidence and trust. This place may already be very familiar to you, or you can just start to imagine a place where you feel safe and at ease. Perhaps this is a place in nature, or a particular room in a house. Take a moment now to go right to that place and notice what you see. Just relax in that safe place and enjoy it for a moment now...

Good.

And when surges begin and when any decisions need to be made, you do this with confidence. You are calm and prepared. Throughout your induction you can choose to close your eyes and go within. You can focus on your breathing and go to your safe place... You are pleasantly surprised at how easy it is to let all noise and activity around you fade away into the background. Notice how good it is to know you don't need to bother to respond to anything at all, unless it is directed specifically to you.

You will be doing hard work, but you've done hard work before and you are capable... There may be times when you feel an intensity like you've never felt before, but this does not surprise you or worry you because you are prepared for this... Instead you choose to notice how easily your mind eases the pressure, letting it spread and flow and dissipate.

You are preparing for all of this ahead of time, training your nervous system to relax so that no matter what eventuality or situation may occur, no matter whether there are delays or surprises, you know you have the freedom to choose to trust and relax. You are always in control...

You use each surge to go deeper into relaxation and trust, each one brings you closer and closer to holding your baby in your arms...

You may notice how easy it is to tune into the smooth rhythm of your relaxed breathing. As you inhale and exhale your chest rises and falls in a comfortable easy rhythm... And as each time you exhale you relax a little more, heavy, loose and limp... sinking deeply into whatever position you are in... Your heartbeat is regular and even throughout your baby's birth... You relax knowing you are going to meet your baby soon.

You easily distract yourself and when you feel a surge begin, without thinking, you deepen into hypnosis... remaining there for as long as the surge lasts...

You know that during a surge you can slowly count down from five to zero and when you reach zero you will be completely relaxed. Five, four, three, two, one, zero and relax.

As soon as each surge finishes this means it's completed and can be forgotten.

Throughout your whole labour, should you need to open your eyes, talk or answer any questions, you will be able to do so while remaining in deep hypnotic relaxation... Any noises you hear from others in the room or outside of the room will not disturb you – instead they are a signal for you to deepen your hypnosis and comfort. Any negative talk in the room becomes white noise to you and just allows you to go deeper into relaxation.

And, even more smoothly than you imagined was possible, your baby is here, placed safely in your arms... Everything went perfectly and you are both doing very well...

You transfer to the postnatal ward and you are relaxed and comfortable... You feel good, knowing all is well...

And now, you are home, safely tucked up in bed with your baby by your side... You are so relaxed and happy. Just enjoy this moment for a while now, enjoy the relief you feel and the joy that your baby is finally here, and you are both home, safe and sound... Now you can look forward to enjoying this special time with your beautiful baby... Just relax, rest and do nothing...

Now bring your thumb and finger together to create a physical cue for these happy, relaxed feelings and any time you want to feel as calm and relaxed as you do now just close your eyes, take a deep breath in and bring your thumb and finger together while breathing out any tension. Do this now – breathe in, and on the relaxing out-breath bring your thumb and finger together... And again, breathe in, and on the out-breath bring your thumb and finger together, creating a cue. And one more time, breathe in and on the relaxing out-breath bring your thumb and finger together... Good.

Every time you listen to this relaxation you find that you relax more and more quickly, easily and deeply. The suggestions become more and more a part of you. They are working more effectively than you can possibly imagine.

And so in a moment or two it will be time to come back to the present knowing you are well prepared for your baby's birth. Bringing all these good feelings of confidence and trust in the staff, in the process and in your decision deep within you, giving you a feeling of peace and calm... And these feelings come much more easily to mind now, whenever you think about your baby's birth... knowing you can recover all these good feelings anytime you choose to do so... And you can take as much of those good feelings with you as you want right now.

And now I'm going to count from one to five and when I get to the number five you will be wide awake and alert, feeling relaxed, refreshed and ready to continue with your day...

If you would like to drift off into a restful, deep sleep, then this is absolutely fine... you will wake up feeling refreshed and relaxed...

Beginning now.

One, starting to become more aware of your body... your fingers... your toes. Two, picturing the room around you now. Three, your eyelids are becoming lighter. Four, feeling more awake and alert. Five, opening your eyes now, completely out of hypnosis, alert, refreshed and ready to continue with your day.

Script 8: General relaxation and confidence (pre- and postnatally)*

You can listen to this confidence-boosting script during pregnancy as well as postnatally.

Take a moment to make yourself comfortable... rest and relax... Close your eyes... Start to become aware of the sensations in your body... Adjust your position to make sure you are sitting completely at ease...

Any sounds you hear outside or in the room can fade away into the background, where it no longer matters... You may notice your breathing... just allow your breathing to be comfortable and steady... Allow any thoughts that appear in your mind to float away, like puffs of clouds... you don't have to think of anything in particular right now so let any thoughts come in and then pass on by... Relax... rest and do nothing...

So as you rest there with your eyes closed know that in a few moments you can sink into a deep hypnotic relaxation... where you find that positive thoughts and feelings flow easily and naturally... where your imagination can become stronger and focused on the positive ideas and suggestions that you will hear... where you can relax easily... Good.

Now open your eyes and without moving your head turn your gaze upwards, this is your hypnotic induction point. Gazing upwards like this makes your eyes feel tired. You can help by imagining that your eyes feel increasingly heavy, and telling yourself they want to close. When your eyes close, let yourself relax completely and continue relaxing...

In a moment, I'm going to begin counting back from ten all the way down to zero. As I count, count down with me in your mind... Imagine with each number we count that your eyes feel more heavy, tired, and

* Scripts 8, 9 and 10 courtesy UK College of Hypnosis and Hypnotherapy. **www. ukhypnosis.com**

sleepy. Let them close just as soon as they want to close...

Beginning now... Ten... drift deeper, Nine... drift deeper, Eight... drift deeper... Seven... drift deeper... Six... drift deeper... Five... drift deeper.... Four... drift deeper..... Three... drift deeper..... Two... drift deeper... One... drift deeper... and zero... let your eyes close all the way down and relax completely... And again... zero... Sleep deeper... Let go and relax completely... Relax your eyes completely... Relax your face completely... Relax your body completely... Relax your mind completely... Just rest and let go.

Good. Now take a breath in and out, releasing any remaining tension on the out-breath. Let go and relax completely now... Just rest as all tension drains away... draining away now just like the grains of fine sand in an hour glass...

You're now growing so deeply relaxed... and your mind is becoming so responsive... and so receptive that everything I now suggest to you is sinking so deeply into your mind... and making a deep and lasting an impression there... taking root permanently and effectively...

During this deep hypnotic relaxation you are going to feel physically stronger and healthier in every way... You are beginning to feel more confident... Every day your mind grows calmer and clearer... more peaceful... more tranquil... You are now able to think more clearly, to see things in their true perspective in a healthy and balanced way... to concentrate more easily... And many good things will continue to happen to you... every day...

Every day... you now grow more emotionally calm... much more settled... much more contented... both mentally and physically... And as you become... more relaxed... each day you now develop much more confidence in yourself... more confidence in your ability to do things... not only in what you have to do each day... but confidence in whatever you wish to do or imagine yourself doing...

And as all these things continue to happen... exactly as I say they are happening... more and more rapidly... powerfully... and completely... with each moment that passes... you grow much happier... much more contented... much more optimistic in every way. You now become much more able to believe in yourself... to rely upon yourself... to trust yourself... to trust your own efforts... your own judgement...and your own opinions.

And you realise that you don't need to be stressed – you can be calm – relaxed – and comfortable – So wonderfully calm and relaxed and comfortable... You much prefer to feel calm, relaxed and comfortable...

Now, in a moment, I'll begin repeating a simple, powerful affirmation which reinforces all of those positive ideas. Listen to the words... 'Every day, I now feel more peace, strength, and confidence...'

Every time I repeat those words that suggestion is penetrating two times deeper into your mind, creating a more powerful, beneficial and lasting transformation in your feelings and behaviour.

Beginning now...

'Every day, I now feel more peace, strength, and confidence...'

[Repeat slowly five times]

Good... Now, in a moment, I'm going to begin counting from one all the way up to five, bringing you out of hypnosis... And you will bring back with you all of those wonderful feelings and keep them with you – remembering them whenever you need to – whenever you want to... Taking the many positive ideas and suggestions you have absorbed into form as new beliefs, new behaviour and new feelings... Taking these new beliefs, and positive feelings into a living reality in your life – and these many positive ideas and feelings grow stronger and more beneficial with each day that passes...

And with each number I count, you are now emerging from hypnosis feeling good. With each number I count you feel better and better, you feel wonderfully good. Peaceful and relaxed.

Beginning now.

One, starting to become more aware of your body, your fingers... your toes. Two, picturing the room around you now. Three, your eyelids are becoming lighter. Four, feeling more awake and alert. Five, opening your eyes now, completely out of hypnosis, alert, refreshed and ready to continue with your day.

Script 9: Leaves on the stream

This is a cognitive diffusion (which is an offshoot of mindfulness) meditation. Cognitive diffusion (or cognitive distancing) is the act of mentally separating yourself from your thoughts and becoming more mindful of the continuous stream of thoughts we have. It's not about changing your thoughts, it's about not getting caught up or swept away with your thoughts, which aren't facts, and instead stepping back and being the non-judgemental observer of them, letting them come in and letting them go. Viewing our thoughts just as thoughts, so we have less entanglement with problematic thoughts. Getting us out of our head and in the present moment. You can listen to this a few times until it is familiar to you, then use it each day or whenever you feel the need to.

Visualise yourself sitting or standing beside a gently flowing stream or river with leaves floating along the surface of the water...

For the next few minutes, take each thought that enters your mind – distance from it and place it on a leaf... let it float by. Do this with each thought – pleasurable, uncomfortable, or neutral. Even if you have happy thoughts, become aware of them, step back from them, place them on a leaf and let them float by...

If your thoughts momentarily cease then continue to watch the stream. Sooner or later, thoughts will tend start up again...

Allow the stream to flow at its own pace. Don't try to speed it up and rush the thoughts along. You're not trying to rush the leaves along or 'get rid of thoughts' or have an empty mind and perfect concentration. You are allowing thoughts to come and go at their own pace – and give them no particular attention...

If your mind says 'I can't do this,' or 'I'm bored,' or 'I'm not doing this right' – then simply step back from those thoughts, detach from them and place those thoughts on leaves, too, and let them pass...

If a leaf gets stuck, allow it to hang around until it's ready to float by. If the thought comes up again, watch it float by another time...

If a difficult or painful feeling arises, simply acknowledge it. Say to yourself, 'I'm aware of having a feeling of boredom/impatience/ frustration/sadness/fear/anger.' Place those thoughts on leaves and allow them to float along...

From time to time, thoughts may hook you and distract you from being fully present in this exercise. This is entirely normal – just as soon as you realise that you've wandered into your thoughts then gently bring your attention back to the exercise. Generally this loss of self-awareness as we become hooked by thoughts becomes less – and we become more and more quickly aware of what we are thinking...

I will be quiet for a moment now to allow you to continue...

Now gently start to bring your attention back to your breath... Take a couple of deep, relaxed breaths and without opening your eyes, bring your awareness back to your body... In your mind's eye picture the room around you... Feel the weight of your body... And now slowly, slowly open your eyes with the intention of carrying this mindfulness with you throughout the rest of the day.

Script 10: Short mindfulness exercise

Step one: mindfulness of the here and now

Pause for a few moments to become more mindful of yourself. Notice how you're currently using your body and your mind, right now, in the present moment. Take a step back from your thoughts and allow yourself to acknowledge and accept any unpleasant feelings you might be having, such as tension, pain, or anxiety... Be aware of yourself as the detached observer of your thoughts and feelings...

Throughout life you've experienced literally millions of different thoughts and feelings and observed many different things. Your current thoughts and feelings are transient, just what you happen to be experiencing right now, sooner or later your attention will move on to other things, and then sometimes it may return to these experiences again.

For now, just be aware of what you're currently experiencing, from moment to moment, without evaluating it, analysing it, or interpreting it. You can have your eyes open or closed, be standing or sitting, it really doesn't matter... Just allow yourself to pause and become mindful of your experience for a few moments. If your mind wanders, that's fine, just acknowledge the fact and bring your awareness patiently back to the exercise you're doing...

Step two: grounding attention in the breathing

Now gradually narrow your focus of attention on to the sensations of your breathing. Don't try to change your breathing, don't try to stop it from changing, just breathe naturally. Accept what your breathing feels like and make room for it to do whatever it wants, let go of any desire to change or control it. Notice the sensations of your breathing, the rise and fall of your belly, perhaps movements in your chest, or even your shoulders. Become aware of even the smallest sensations that accompany your breathing, feelings you may not have noticed before. Keep paying attention to your breathing to help ground your attention in the reality of the present moment.

If you're aware of any unpleasant feelings anywhere in your body, just allow yourself to accept them patiently and let them come and go as they please, or to remain the same. Let go completely of any struggle against them and instead study them from a more detached perspective... Combine awareness of the breath with awareness of the body by imagining your breath continually passing right through that part of your body where the unpleasant feelings are happening... Use your breath to centre your attention on that part of your body for a while. As you breathe in and out, continue to actively accept those sensations and allow yourself to fully experience them. Let go completely of any struggle against them. Make room for the feelings to run their course, or come and go freely by imagining a sense of space opening up around them. You are not your breath, you are not those sensations, you are not your emotions or even your thoughts; you're the detached observer of all of these things, viewing experiences from a distance as they come and go without struggle.

Step three: expanding awareness throughout the body

Now gradually begin to expand your awareness beyond those sensations. Continue to be aware of your breathing and any part of your body that you've been attending to but, in addition, allow your awareness to begin spreading through the rest of your body, throughout the trunk of your body, your arms, your legs, your neck and head. Become aware of your whole body as one, and continue to accept any unpleasant sensations you're experiencing, but also begin to notice what else you're experiencing, more and more, progressively widening the sphere of your attention. Not trying to avoid or control unpleasant experiences but rather expanding beyond them.

Now gradually spread your awareness out further beyond your body and into the room around you, where you are and what you're doing right now. Continue to notice how you're using your body and mind as you look slowly around you. As you finish the exercise and begin interacting with the external world and perhaps other people, take that sense of mindfulness and self-awareness with you into your environment and any tasks at hand. If you continue to notice any unpleasant sensations, that's fine, just accept them, let go of any struggle against them, and gently expand your attention beyond them to the world around you and the way you're interacting with life as you move into action.

References and further reading

Third stage of labour

Active versus expectant management for women in the third stage of labour – a Cochrane Systematic Review published: 13 February 2019. www.cochranelibrary.com/cdsr/doi/10.1002/14651858.CD007412.pub5/full

Effect of Spontaneous Pushing Versus Valsalva Pushing in the Second Stage of Labour on Mother and Fetus: A Systematic Review of Randomised Trials. May 2011. pubmed.ncbi.nlm.nih.gov/21392242

Does Skin-To-Skin Contact and Breast Feeding at Birth Affect the Rate of Primary Postpartum Haemorrhage: Results of a Cohort Study. 2015 Jul 29. pubmed.ncbi.nlm.nih.gov/26277824

www.babycentre.co.uk/x562146/should-i-have-a-managed-or-physiological-third-stage

Home birth/continuity of care/independent midwives

Continuity of care by a primary midwife (caseload midwifery) increases women's satisfaction with antenatal, intrapartum and postpartum care: results from the COSMOS randomised controlled trial. 3rd February 2016. bmcpregnancychildbirth.biomedcentral.com/articles/10.1186/s12884-016-0798-y

Hodnett et al 'Continuous support for women during childbirth, NCBl 2012. www.ncbi.nlm.nih.gov/pubmed/23076901

Midwife-led continuity models of care compared with other models of care for women during pregnancy, birth and early parenting. 28 April 2016. www.cochrane.org/CD004667/PREG_midwife-led-continuity-models-care-compared-other-models-care-women-during-pregnancy-birth-and-early

Continuity of care: what you need to know. September 2017. www.nct.org. uk/pregnancy/who-will-care-for-you-during-pregnancy/continuity-care-what-you-need-know

www.nct.org.uk/labour-birth/deciding-where-give-birth/giving-birth-home/home-births-are-they-safe

Perinatal and maternal outcomes by planned place of birth for healthy women with low risk pregnancies: the Birthplace in England national prospective cohort study. *BMJ* 25 November 2011. www.bmj.com/content/343/bmj.d7400

www.nct.org.uk/labour-birth/deciding-where-give-birth/giving-birth-home/home-births-are-they-safe

Women choosing home birth more likely to breastfeed. *Nursing Times*. 10 August 2016. www.nursingtimes.net/news/research-and-innovation/women-choosing-home-birth-more-likely-to-breastfeed-10-08-2016

Quigley, C., Taut, C., Zigman, T. et al 'Association between home birth and breast feeding outcomes: a cross-sectional study in 28125 mother-infant pairs from Ireland and the UK', *BMJ Open* 2016. doi:10.1136/bmjopen-2015-010551 (Accessed via www.sarawickham.com/research-updates/home-birth-is-significantly-associated-with-breastfeeding)

Place of birth

Choosing where to have your baby: www.nice.org.uk/guidance/cg190/ifp/chapter/Choosing-where-to-have-your-baby

Birthplace in England Research Programme/The Birthplace Study 2011, hwww.npeu.ox.ac.uk/birthplace

Positions for labour

The Evidence on: birthing position. 2 February 2018. evidencebasedbirth.com/evidence-birthing-positions

Mothers' position during the first stage of labour. 9 October 2013. www.cochrane.org/CD003934/PREG_mothers-position-during-the-first-stage-of-labour

Massage

Silva Gallo, R.B., Santana, L.S., Jorge-Ferreira, C.H., et al 'Massage reduced severity of pain during labour: a randomised trial', *J Physiother* 59(2):109-16, 2012. core.ac.uk/download/pdf/82141422.pdf

Effect of Massage Therapy on Duration of Labour: A Randomized Controlled Trial - www.ncbi.nlm.nih.gov/pmc/articles/PMC4866196/#:~:text=conducted%20%5B7%5D.-,Massage%20is%20an%20old%20technique%20that%20is%20widely%20used%20in,contractions%20%5B9%%E2%80%9312%5D.

Aromatherapy/using a scent as a cue

Aromatherapy in Midwifery Practice, Denise Tiran, 2016

Posthypnotic use of olfactory stimulus for pain management: nvvh.com/wp-content/uploads/2015/08/IJCEH-62-2-05.pdf

Hypnotherapeutic Olfactory Conditioning (HOC): Case Studies of Needle Phobia, Panic Disorder, and Combat-Induced PTSD. pubmed.ncbi.nlm.nih.gov/19234966

TENS machines

TENS for pain relief during labour. evidencebasedbirth.com/transcutaneous-electrical-nerve-stimulation-tens-for-pain-relief-during-labor

Pethidine

www.babycentre.co.uk/a542577/pethidine

Doulas

Evidence on: Doulas. 4 May 2019. evidencebasedbirth.com/the-evidence-for-doulas

Visualisation

Your brain on imagination: It's a lot like reality, study shows. December 10, 2018 University of Colorado at Boulder. www.sciencedaily.com/re-leases/2018/12/181210144943.htm

Pain relief – active birth and positions

Position for women during the second stage of labour. elearning.rcog.org.uk//mechanisms-normal-labour-and-birth/practical-management/position-women-during

WHO recommendation on adoption of mobility and upright position

during labour in women at low risk. extranet.who.int/rhl/topics/
preconception-pregnancy-childbirth-and-postpartum-care/care-during-
childbirth/care-during-labour-1st-stage/who-recommendation-adoption-
mobility-and-upright-position-during-labour-women-low-risk

Waterbirth

evidencebasedbirth.com/waterbirth
www.babycentre.co.uk/a542005/what-the-research-says-about-water-birth

Epidurals

Epidurals in labour: what you need to know. www.oaa-anaes.ac.uk/assets/_
managed/editor/File/Info%20for%20Mothers/EIC/2008_eic_english.pdf

Monitoring

The evidence on: monitoring. evidencebasedbirth.com/fetal-monitoring
Fetal Monitoring: Creating a Culture of Safety With Informed Choice.
2013. www.ncbi.nlm.nih.gov/pmc/articles/PMC4010242
Intrapartum care for healthy women and babies. NICE Clinical
guideline CG190. 1.10 Monitoring during labour Measuring fetal
heart rate. 21 February 2017. www.nice.org.uk/guidance/cg190/chapter/
Recommendations#monitoring-during-labour
Monitoring your baby's heartbeat in labour. www.aims.org.uk/information/
item/monitoring-your-babys-heartbeat-in-labour

Assisted birth

The Effect of Epidural Analgesia on the Delivery Outcome of Induced
Labour: A Retrospective Case Series. 20 November 2016. www.ncbi.
nlm.nih.gov/pmc/articles/PMC5136389
Induction of labour in women with normal pregnancies at or beyond
term. 9 May 2018. www.cochrane.org/CD004945/PREG_induction-
labour-women-normal-pregnancies-or-beyond-term

Stitches and healing

Your recovery after birth: Oxford University Hospitals. www.ouh.nhs.uk/

patient-guide/leaflets/files/4895Pchildbirth.pdf

Perineal massage

What Is the Evidence for Perineal Massage During Pregnancy to Prevent Tearing? 18 December 2012. www.lamaze.org/Connecting-the-Dots/ what-is-the-evidence-for-perineal-massage-during-pregnancy-to-prevent-tearing

Induction of labour

AIMS – How accurate is my due date? February 2020. www.aims.org.uk/ information/item/due-date

I'm overdue: now what? www.babycentre.co.uk/a552040/im-overdue-now-what

Labour Induction at Term – How great is the risk of refusing it? www.aims. org.uk/journal/item/induction-at-term

Inducing labour. Clinical guideline [CG70] www.nice.org.uk/guidance/cg70/ chapter/Introduction

Sweeps

Membrane sweeping for induction of labour. www.cochrane.org/ CD000451/PREG_membrane-sweeping-induction-labour

www.nct.org.uk/labour-birth/getting-ready-for-birth/overdue-baby-what-happens-if-my-baby-late#tag-target-4

Breast stimulation

Natural labour induction series: breast stimulation. evidencebasedbirth. com/evidence-using-breast-stimulation-to-naturally-induce-labor/

Caesarean birth

www.cochrane.org/CD011562/PREG_does-chewing-gum-after-caesarean-section-lead-quicker-recovery-functionwithin

The natural caesarean: a woman-centred technique. www.ncbi.nlm.nih. gov/pmc/articles/PMC2613254

Hypnosis

The UK College of Hypnosis and Hypnotherapy. www.ukhypnosis.com

The Science of Self-Hypnosis: The Evidence Based Way to Hypnotise Yourself. Adam Eason, 2013.

Handbook of Hypnotic Suggestions and Metaphors. The American Society of Clinical Hypnosis. Edited by D. Corydon Hammond. 1990

Dick-Read, G. *Childbirth Without Fear*, Pinter & Martin, 2013.

Hypnosis-based Interventions During Pregnancy and Childbirth and Their Impact on Women's Childbirth Experience: A Systematic Review. pubmed.ncbi.nlm.nih.gov/32087396

Mindfulness

Interviews with John Kabat-Zinn on Mindfulness-Based Stress Reduction. www.youtube.com/watch?v=puzAe4G6uDw

General pregnancy and/or postnatal topics

www.nct.org.uk

www.babycentre.co.uk

www.kickscount.org.uk

The Baby Buddy app is targeted at younger parents, aged between 16 and 24 www.bestbeginnings.org.uk/baby-buddy

Birth research and information

www.sarawickham.com

www.aims.org.uk

www.evidencebasedbirth.com

www.midwifethinking.com

Your rights in birth/support with your choices

www.birthrights.org.uk

www.aims.org.uk

PALS – the Patient Advisory & Liaison Service (based at each UK Hospital)

Positive Birth Support

www.positivebirthmovement.org
www.tellmeagoodbirthstory.com

Evidence-based guidelines for the UK

www.nice.org.uk
www.nice.org.uk/guidance/cg190?unlid=46050102020 163113029

Breastfeeding help

Books

The Positive Breastfeeding Book by Amy Brown (Pinter & Martin)
You've Got It In You, a Positive Guide to Breastfeeding by Emma Pickett
  (Matador)
The Microbiome Effect by Toni Harman and Alex Wakeford (Pinter &
  Martin)

Alcohol and breastfeeding
www.breastfeedingnetwork.org.uk/alcohol/
www.laleche.org.uk/alcohol-and-breastfeeding/

Benefits of breastfeeding

www.nct.org.uk/baby-toddler/feeding/early-days/benefits-breastfeeding

Cluster feeding

kellymom.com/parenting/parenting-faq/fussy-evening

Engorgement

www.laleche.org.uk/engorged-breasts-avoiding-and-treating

Expressing

abm.me.uk/breastfeeding-information/expressing-breast-milk

Finger feeding supplementary feeds

breastfeeding.support/what-is-finger-feeding
www.ouh.nhs.uk/patient-guide/leaflets/files/11016Pfingerfeeding.pdf

Formula feeding

www.firststepsnutrition.org/parents-carers
www.unicef.org.uk/babyfriendly/baby-friendly-resources/bottle-feeding-
    resources/infant-formula-responsive-bottle-feeding-guide-for-parents/
www.unicef.org.uk/babyfriendly/wp-content/uploads/sites/2/2008/02/
    start4life_guide_to_bottle_-feeding.pdf

Harvesting colostrum

www.babycentre.co.uk/x25024458/should-i-harvest-my-colostrum-before-my-
    baby-is-born

Milk supply

www.theboobgeek.com/blog/making-enough-breastmilk.html
www.theboobgeek.com/blog/oversupply-too-much-of-a-good-thing.html

Nursing bras

www.babycentre.co.uk/a562823/buying-a-nursing-bra

Partner's role

www.nct.org.uk/sites/default/files/related_documents/
    partnersAndBreastfeeding_web.pdf

Positioning and attachment

www.breastfeeding.asn.au/bfinfo/attachment-breast
globalhealthmedia.org/portfolio-items/attaching-your-baby-at-the-breast
www.emmasdiary.co.uk/baby/breastfeeding/breastfeeding-positions-for-mums

Relactation

www.llli.org/breastfeeding-info/relactation

Skin-to-skin

www.laleche.org.uk/whats-big-deal-skin-skin

Tongue-tie

www.laleche.org.uk/tongue-tie

Troubleshooting

www.babycentre.co.uk/c545887/breastfeeding-problems-and-solutions

Seeking support

www.breastfeedingnetwork.org.uk/breastfeeding-support
www.nhs.uk/start4life/baby/breastfeeding/breastfeeding-help-and-support/
www.nct.org.uk/baby-toddler/feeding/early-days/how-find-breastfeeding-
    support-your-area-when-you-need-it

Weaning

www.nhs.uk/start4life/weaning
www.essentialparent.com/lesson/ten-laid-back-steps-to-giving-your-baby-
    solid-foods-by-dr-amy-brown-16313

Independent Midwives and Doulas

www.imuk.org.uk
www.doula.org.uk

Mental health/pre and postnatal depression support

www.pandasfoundation.org.uk
www.mind.org.uk

Social

mumsmeetup.com
mummysocial.com
letsmush.com
www.babycentre.co.uk/a1006203/mums-tips-how-to-meet-other-new-mums

Acknowledgements

Thank you to all the authors, websites, researchers and academics for such a wonderful body of evidence and research for me to draw upon when writing this book. I also thank all of those who kindly reviewed and read through the book in its draft format. I offer many grateful thanks to you all.

Special thanks go to Sue Sawyer and Mark Davis of the UK College of Hypnosis and Hypnotherapy which can be found at www.ukhypnosis.com.

I am especially grateful to Kate Cameron who has contributed chapter 20 on breastfeeding.

Index

Notes